Multifunctional Proteins: Catalytic/Structural and Regulatory

Editor

James F. Kane, Ph. D.
Senior Scientist
Monsanto Company
St. Louis, Missouri

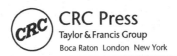

CRC Press
Taylor & Francis Group
Boca Raton London New York

CRC Press is an imprint of the
Taylor & Francis Group, an **informa** business

CRC Press
Taylor & Francis Group
6000 Broken Sound Parkway NW, Suite 300
Boca Raton, FL 33487-2742

Reissued 2019 by CRC Press

© 1983 by Taylor & Francis Group, LLC
CRC Press is an imprint of Taylor & Francis Group, an Informa business

No claim to original U.S. Government works

A Library of Congress record exists under LC control number:

Publisher's Note
The publisher has gone to great lengths to ensure the quality of this reprint but points out that some imperfections in the original copies may be apparent.

Disclaimer
The publisher has made every effort to trace copyright holders and welcomes correspondence from those they have been unable to contact.

ISBN 13: 978-0-367-22816-3 (hbk)
ISBN 13: 978-0-367-22817-0 (pbk)
ISBN 13: 978-0-429-27700-9 (ebk)

Visit the Taylor & Francis Web site at http://www.taylorandfrancis.com and the
CRC Press Web site at http://www.crcpress.com

PREFACE

The term multifunctional protein conjures up many images. Allosteric enzymes, for example, can be viewed as possessing two cellular functions, one catalytic and one regulatory. Other proteins, such as transaminases, have been described as multifunctional because their ambiguous substrate requirements allow for multiple catalytic functions albeit at the same catalytic site. In a similar fashion, we perceived the aminotransferase subunit G from *Bacillus subtilis* as a multifunctional protein because it took part in two distinct biochemical pathways. Although it is easy to see the utility of such proteins in cellular metabolism and biochemical evolution, one could argue about their multifunctionality. A strict definition of multifunctional proteins has been proposed by K. Kirschner and H. Bisswanger, in *Annu. Rev. Biochem.*, 1977, and defines these proteins as being composed of a single polypeptide, or a polymeric enzyme complex, possessing more than one autonomous catalytic and/or binding site. Theoretically, these sites can be measured independently of one another. With this definition, the allosteric proteins and enzymes with ambiguous catalytic functions are not multifunctional. Included in this definition, however, would be (1) the subunit G protein of *B. subtilis,* since it possesses binding sites for glutamine and two other proteins, and (2) a vast array of proteins that clearly possess autonomous domains on a single polypeptide chain or enzyme complex. In between these two extremes, however, lies an equally fascinating group of proteins that demonstrate multiple cellular functions, one of which is regulatory. In many cases it is not clear if these latter proteins fit the strict definition of multifunctional proteins by possessing independently measurable autonomous domains. Nevertheless, the multiple roles these proteins appear to play in cellular metabolism suggest that, when all the results are compiled, these proteins may be called multifunctional. I am reminded of a quote attributed to an Oriental Proverb: "When the dust passes thou wilt see whether thou ridest a horse or an ass." Regardless of the outcome of my projection, it is increasingly clear that proteins containing catalytic/structural and regulatory functions serve an important role in cellular metabolism. An understanding of this group of enzymes can only serve to increase our appreciation of the multitude of cellular control mechanisms.

THE EDITOR

James F. Kane, Ph.D., received his undergraduate degree from St. Joseph's University in June of 1964. After one year of graduate work at the Biology Department of St. Louis University, he completed a Ph.D. degree in Biology, with emphasis on cellular physiology and biochemistry, at the State University of New York at Buffalo in February, 1969.

Dr. Kane received an NIH Postdoctoral Fellowship (1968-70) and pursued studies in microbial physiology and biochemistry with Dr. Roy A. Jensen at the Department of Microbiology of Baylor College of Medicine in Houston, Texas. He subsequently took a position in the Department of Microbiology at the University of Tennessee Center for Health Sciences, and remained at UTCHS until June, 1980.

Presently Dr. Kane is a Senior Research Specialist in the Corporate Research Laboratories of Monsanto Company in St. Louis, Missouri. He is a member of the American Society for Microbiology and the Federation of Biological Chemists. His research interests include the evolution of multifunctional proteins and their role in regulation of cellular activity.

ACKNOWLEDGMENTS

I would like to thank the contributors of this volume for their patience and participation in this effort, and Milton H. Saier for his contribution of the quote from Homer — *The Iliad*.

"The Chimaera was held to be unconquerable. She was a most singular portent, a thing of immortal make, not human, lion fronted and snake behind, a goat in the middle, and snorting out the breath of the terrible flame of bright fire."

Homer, *The Iliad*.

CONTRIBUTORS

Jean E. Brenchley
Research Director
Genex Corporation
Gaithersburg, Maryland

Daniel H. Doherty
Research Associate
M.C.D.B.
University of Colorado
Boulder, Colorado

Peter Gauss
Research Associate
M.C.D.B. Biology
University of Colorado
Boulder, Colorado

Larry Gold
Professor
M.C.D.B. Biosciences
University of Colorado
Boulder, Colorado

James F. Kane, Ph.D.
Senior Scientist
Montsanto Company
St. Louis, Missouri

John E. Leonard
Postdoctoral Fellow
Cancer Center
University of California at San Diego
La Jolla, California

Rolf Menzel
National Institutes of Health
Bethesda, Maryland

Masayasu Nomura, Ph.D.
Professor
Institute for Enzyme Research
University of Wisconsin
Madison, Wisconsin

Milton Saier, Ph.D.
Professor
Department of Biology
University of California at San Diego
La Jolla, California

Rudolph Spangler
Faculty Fellow
Department of Biological Sciences
Columbia University
New York, New York

John Yates, Ph.D.
Post-doctorate
McArdle Laboratory for Cancer Research
University of Wisconsin
Madison, Wisconsin

Geoffrey Zubay
Professor
Department of Biological Sciences
Columbia University
New York, New York

TABLE OF CONTENTS

Chapter 1

INTRODUCTION

James F. Kane

TABLE OF CONTENTS

I. PERSPECTIVES ON REGULATION

The whole of cellular metabolism can be viewed as a highly branched and extremely complex metabolic pathway. Molecular activities within the cell are fine-tuned to incorporate inorganic and organic materials into the building blocks for cellular growth. For the most part these cellular activities are tightly regulated, and complex interlocking regulatory circuits provide a proper balance of end products for optimal cell growth. Indeed, the orderly developments in cellular differentiation are the result of such regulatory mechanisms exerted at the level of enzyme activity or gene expression. In the former case, enzyme activity is regulated by effector molecules that serve to enhance or inhibit activity. These molecules generally are structurally distinct from the substrates and bind to the enzymes at sites other than the catalytic sites, that is, at allosteric sites. In the latter case, enzyme activity is regulated by controlling the amount of enzyme synthesized, and this can be accomplished at the level of either gene transcription or translation.

The elegant studies of Jacob and Monod[1] on the lactose operon of *Escherichia coli* illustrated a simple yet effective means for the control of gene expression. In this system, the protein product of a regulatory gene, (i), binds to a region of the DNA called the operator locus (o). This protein prevents transcription of the structural genes of the lactose operon by the RNA polymerase that is bound to the DNA at a site called the promoter (p). This repressor protein, however, also possesses a binding site for a small molecule, namely β-allolactose. When β-allolactose binds to the repressor protein the protein-allolactose complex no longer interacts with the operator region of the DNA and the structural genes of the lactose operon are transcribed into mRNA by the RNA polymerase. This type of control is called induction and the "i" gene product is called a negative effector because it functions only in stopping synthesis of mRNA from the DNA. Subsequent studies have shown that the regulation of the lactose operon is more complex and involves cyclic AMP and a cyclic AMP binding protein.[2] These latter elements are essential for the efficient transcription of the lactose operon by RNA polymerase and are, therefore, called positive regulatory elements. Despite this added level of complexity the role of the lactose repressor protein remains unchanged from the original description of its function by Jacob and Monod. That is, its sole function is the negative control, or turning off, of the transcription of the lactose operon. In this case, the regulatory gene "i" is itself constitutively expressed: that is, its expression is not regulated.[3]

The Jacob-Monod model of the control of gene expression has been applied to many operons. Despite the simplicity of this model and the fact that *E. coli* uses this mechanism to control the *lac* operon effectively, it has become increasingly clear that *E. coli* and other organisms have utilized many different mechanisms to regulate gene transcription and control cellular activity. In 1964 Maas and McFall[4] suggested an alternate explanation to the independent repressor protein such as the "i" gene product of the *lac* operon. In their hypothesis the first enzyme of a metabolic sequence would function both as a catalytic protein and as a regulator of gene expression. Since it had already been demonstrated that the first enzyme was the site for feedback inhibition by the end-product of the pathway, the allosteric enzyme was proposed also to function in a regulatory manner by preventing gene transcription or translation. The regulation of gene expression by the product of that gene is called autogenous[5,6] or autoregulation.[7] From the point of view of cellular economy this concept is most attractive. The cell is freed from producing proteins, whose sole function is to regulate gene expression as was found for the lactose repressor. Despite the seeming advantage of such a system, the prevalence of this type of regulatory mechanism has been limited. In an excellent review, Savageau[8] presents theoretical and experimental data on the types of autogenously regulated systems and compares these to the classically (i.e., monofunctional repressor as the "i" gene product of the *lac* operon) regulated systems. These autogenously regulated proteins would of necessity be multifunctional from the point of view of cellular metabolism.

II. DEFINITION OF MULTIFUNCTIONAL PROTEINS

Multifunctional proteins have been defined as proteins composed of a single polypeptide or multienzyme complexes possessing more than one autonomous catalytic and/or binding site.[9] These sites must constitute discrete domains on the individual protein subunit or the multimeric complex of subunits. In previous reviews on this topic,[9,10] a number of well defined proteins have been described but none of these proteins, save one, served a regulatory function. The sole regulatory protein described was the lactose repressor. Although this protein possesses two distinct binding sites for the operator DNA and the small molecule inducer, it serves only one cellular function, namely, repression of transcription.

In this book we describe a very interesting class of proteins that clearly possess multiple cellular functions (Table 1). Within this class there are proteins that function as: (a) catalytic and regulatory molecules, (b) structural and regulatory molecules, and (c) dual regulatory molecules. Although the exclusiveness of the distinct domains on these molecules is not unequivocally proven with a large number of these proteins, preliminary results are consistent with including them in the above definition. Many of these proteins may be autogenously regulated, although this is not a prerequisite for their classification as multifunctional proteins.

III. CATALYTIC/REGULATORY PROTEINS

In ascribing a regulatory function to a catalytic protein it is necessary to distinguish these functions genetically, biochemically, and biophysically. The most rigorous experimental data are obtained by measuring the discrete binding activities of the protein(s) involved. This, of course, is also the most difficult task requiring homogeneous protein preparations and the appropriate reagents, or substrates, to assess the binding and catalytic functions. Genetic methods offer a powerful alternative in the study of multifunctional proteins in that highly purified protein preparations are not needed. Some caution, however, must be exercised to avoid the overinterpretation of these results. Although a mutation at the catalytic site of a protein might affect its regulatory function, it must be determined that such aberations in regulation are not the result of either mutations in closely linked regulatory genes or a physiological consequence of decreased enzymatic activity. In addition, when the catalytic and regulatory sites are autonomous, one should be able to genetically alter each site independently.

Some examples of enzymes that appear to have both catalytic and regulatory roles in cellular metabolism are shown in Table 1. Of these examples, mannitol enzyme II from *E. coli*, proline oxidase from *Salmonella typhimurum*,[12] and RNA polymerase from *E. coli*[13] are described in detail in later chapters of this book. The multifunctional nature of the remaining examples has been verified to varying degrees and will only be briefly described. It is assumed, but not proven, that the different activities occur at discrete sites on these proteins.

Responsible for the acylation of amino acids to the cognate tRNA are tRNA synthetases. Recently, Putney and Schimmel[14] demonstrated that alanine tRNA synthetase also served a regulatory role in the cell. This protein bound specifically to a palindromic sequence flanking the promoter sites of the *alaS* gene which specifies the alanine tRNA synthetase. This binding, that was enhanced by alanine but not other amino acids, affected the transcription of the *alaS* gene in vitro and was proposed to be a repressor of its own synthesis. These authors also propose that this regulatory mechanism is of general significance for other tRNA synthetases.

TABLE 1

| Protein | Functions | | Source | Ref. |
	Catalytic/Structural	Regulatory		
Catalytic				
Mannitol enzyme II	Mannitol receptor kinase and transport	Autoregulatory	*E. coli*	11
Proline oxidase	Proline degradation transport	Autoregulatory	*S. typhimurium*	12
$\beta\beta'$	RNA polymerase	Autoregulatory	*E. coli*	13
Ala-tRNA synthetase	Acylation of alanine	Autoregulatory	*E. coli*	14
α-Subunit of tryptophan synthase	Tryptophon biosynthesis	Autoregulatory	*P. putida*	15
recA Gene product	Protease; binds single strand DNA; recombination	Autoregulatory	*E. coli*	18—24
himA gene product	Site specific recombination	Autoregulatory	*E. coli*	25
Dihydrofolate reductase	Synthesis of tetrahydrofolate	Autoregulatory	*Streptococcus pneumoniae*	26
	Synthesis of tetrahydrofolate	Autoregulatory	*Bacillus subtilis*	27—29
Glutamine synthetase	Synthesis of glutamine	Control of nitrogen metabolism	*Enterobacteriaceae*	30
Threonine, deaminase	Biosyntheses of isoleucine	Autoregulatory	*Salmonella typhimurium* *Sacchromyces cerevislae*	31—35 37
Nitrate reductase	Reduction of NO_3^- to NO_2^-	Regulates NO_3^- reductive pathway Autoregulatory	*Aspergillus nidulans*	41—42
Structural				
Ribosomal proteins	Ribosome structure	Autoregulatory	*E. coli*	51
S_{10}	Ribosome structure	Transcription termination	*E. coli*	52
Gene 32 product	Binds single stranded DNA	Autoregulatory	T_4 phage	53
Scaffolding protein	Assembles phage coat	Autoregulatory	P_{22} Phage	54
T-antigen	Initiation of DNA synthesis Late gene transcription	Autoregulatory	SV40	55
Ad DNA binding protein	Binds single stranded DNA	Autoregulatory	Adenovirus	57
Regulatory				
hut Repressor	None	Autoregulatory regulates *hut* operon	*S. typhimurium*	60
AraC gene product	None	Autoregulatory regulate *araBAD* operon	*E. coli*	61
Tn_3 repressor	None	Autoregulatory regulates translocation	*E. coli*	62
lexA Gene product	None	Autoregulatory regulates *recA* regulates other SOS functions	*E. coli*	63 and 64

TABLE 1 (continued)

Protein	Catalytic/Structural	Functions Regulatory	Source	Ref.
tyrR Gene product	None	Autoregulatory Regulates at least six operons involved in aromatic amino acid synthesis and transport	*E. coli*	65

Tryptophan synthase, the last enzyme in the tryptophan biosynthetic pathway, has been found to be autogenously controlled in *Pseudomonas putida*.[15] This enzyme is composed of two subunits specified by the *trpAB* genes. In *P. putida*, these two genes form their own operon.[16] Proctor and Crawford[15,17] demonstrated that the *trpAB* operon is induced by indole glycerol phosphate and that the α subunit of tryptophan synthase (the product of the *trpA* gene) is an integral part of the regulatory mechanism controlling the expression of the *trpAB* operon. Regulatory mutations outside the *trpAB* cluster and alterations in the pool levels of small molecule effectors have been ruled out, but it is not clear how the *trpA* gene product functions in gene control.

Another interesting multifunctional protein is the so-called "Protein X" or the *recA* gene product of *E. coli*. This protein has the following properties: protease activity[18-20] catalyzes the formation of D loops, that is, binding of a single stranded DNA molecule to its homologous counterpart in a double stranded DNA molecule,[21,22] binding and hydrolysis of ATP,[18-22] and association with membrane.[23,24] Although the molecular basis for the many functions of the *recA* protein are largely unknown, the regulatory function of the *recA* protein appears to be related to its protease activity. That is, the *recA* gene product controls its own synthesis by proteolytically degrading the repressor protein synthesized by the *lexA* gene. This mechanism of autogenous control is unique among those proposed in this volume where control appears to be at the level of gene transcription or translation.

An additional component of the SOS system in *E. coli* is the product of the *himA* gene.[25] This protein appears to be a subunit (α) of the integration host factor (IHF) required for site specific recombination and is a necessary component for the integration of λ into the DNA. It is also needed for the efficient expression of the *int* and *CI* genes of λ. Miller et al.,[25] report that the *himA* gene product also serves two regulatory roles; namely, it is a negative repressor of its own synthesis and it represses the *himD* gene that specifies the β subunit of IHF. The control of *himA* appears to be complex since mutations that induce the SOS system, that is, *recA* or *lexA* mutations, also induce the *himA* gene. Although the relationship between IHF and the *lexA* gene product is not clear, mutations in *himA* and *lexA* do not appear to be additive in affecting expression from the *himA* gene.

Sirotnak and his co-workers[26] have isolated a spontaneous amethopterin resistant mutant of *Diplococcus pneumoniae*. The mutant had a defect in the structural gene and simultaneously overproduced dihydrofolate reductase. Since the mutation was spontaneous it is unlikely that both the structural gene and an independent regulatory gene were altered. It has not been established, however, that dihydrofolate reductase binds to DNA carrying the *dfr* gene and controls its transcription or binds to *dfr* specific RNA and controls translation. Additionally, it is not clear if the resultant changes in enzyme level reflect altered pool levels of regulatory effectors. In a similar study we have isolated spontaneous trimethoprim resistant mutants of *Bacillus subtilis* that contain altered dihydrofolate reductase.[27] Three classes of resistance were identified.

The first class (T2) contained a dihydrofolate reductase that had an increased resistance to the inhibitor trimethoprim as well as an increase in the overall enzyme activity. We have not proven that the increased activity resulted from an increased rate of gene transcription, however. In the second class (TTK24), the inhibitory effects of trimethoprim on enzyme activity were markedly decreased but the enzyme activity was not affected. The final class of mutants (T7) contained a markedly increased activity for dihydrofolate reductase with no change in the trimethoprim sensitivity of this enzyme. At the present time the *dfr* genes from these various classes either have been or will be cloned and are under study.[28,29]

There have been reports that implicate multiple functions for other catalytic enzymes, but recent results suggest that, if these proteins were to play a regulatory role, then it would be a secondary or modifying one. First, glutamine synthetase has been proposed to be an important control element in its own transcription as well as in genes involved in nitrogen metabolism. Many of these results, however, could be explained by mutations in loci tightly linked to *glnA*, the structural gene for glutamine synthetase. This topic is addressed in detail in this volume.[30]

Second, original studies on the *ilv EDS operon*[31] suggested that threonine deaminase (the product of *ilvA* gene) was a key regulatory element in the control of this operon. However, deletion of the *ilvA* region in *E. coli* did not significantly affect the regulation of the remaining genes.[32] There are several points worth noting that support a role, albeit secondary, for threonine deaminase in regulation: (1) no regulatory gene has been identified that affects the *ilvEDS* operon;[33] (2) several mutations affecting regulation appear to be in the *ilvA* gene;[33] (3) the *ilv* operon contains an attenuator region,[34-35] a site known to exert a regulatory control[36] in response to acylated or unacylated tRNA; (4) threonine deaminase has been shown to bind leucyl-tRNA^{Leu};[31] and (5) there is evidence that threonine deaminase may be a positive regulatory element in *Sacchromyces cerevisiae*.[37]

Third, the histidine operon from *Salmonella typhimurium* does not appear to have a separate regulatory gene that controls transcription or translation. Goldberger and his co-workers[38] had suggested that the first enzyme of the histidine pathway, the product of the first gene *(hisG)* in the operon, was autoregulatory. Again, this gene product does not serve a primary role in regulation[39] although a secondary function at the attenuator site[40] cannot be excluded.

Fourth, in *Aspergillus nidulans* nitrate reductase, the first enzyme in the nitrate assimilatory pathway has been reported to control several loci involved in this complex pathway.[41,42]

Finally, a glutamine amidotransferase subunit, designated subunit G, has been found to be common to two different biosynthetic pathways in *B. subtilis*[43] and *Acinetobacter calcoaceticus*.[44] In *B. subtilis*, subunit G binds to subunit A to constitute *p*-aminobenzoate[45] synthase that participates in the synthesis of folate, and to subunit E to constitute anthranilate synthase, the first enzyme specific to the biosynthesis of tryptophan.[46] The AG and EG complexes can utilize glutamine as the amide donor whereas subunits A and E cannot. Mutations in subunit G affect glutamine dependent amidation but not the binding to at least subunit E.[47] It has been proposed that subunit G may function in other biochemical amidotransferase reactions and that the *trpG* locus is subject to autoregulation.[45] Neither of these hypotheses have been proven, however. It is clear that there are at least three binding sites on subunit G for glutamine, subunit A, and subunit E. Other multifunctional proteins within the tryptophan pathway have been found[48,49] but none of these appear to serve a primary regulatory role.[50]

IV. STRUCTURAL/REGULATORY PROTEINS

Several structural proteins have also been found to serve regulatory roles in cellular metabolism. Six examples of such proteins are illustrated in Table 1.

Ribosomal proteins are intimately involved with the structure of the large and small ribosomal subunits. The autoregulatory role of these proteins is illustrated in a later chapter.[51]

Another example of regulation by a ribosomal protein has also been described.[52] Friedman et al.[52] propose that the S10 protein of the small ribosome of *E. coli* plays a role in transcription termination. The basis for this hypothesis involves a mutation in the locus that specifies the S10 protein that prevents phage λ from replicating. Their model proposes that the S10 protein interacts with the λ N gene product and prevents antitermination. The mechanism for the S10 protein's role in termination of the RNA polymerase is unknown.

Several phage and viral proteins have been found to possess multiple functions one of which is regulatory. The gene 32 product in phage T_4 is described in detail later[53] and will not be further discussed.

In phage P22, a protein, called the scaffolding protein (P8), is responsible for assembling approximately 420 molecules of the viral coat protein to form a prohead shell.[54] Amber mutations within gene 8, that specifies the 42,000 dalton P8 protein, result in the loss of prohead formation. Additional studies with various phage mutants suggest that the level of P8 produced is directly proportional to the free P8 inside the cell. That is, with mutants blocked in the packaging of DNA, P8 is trapped in the prohead shell and the synthesis of P8 is increased. This evidence is used to support the concept that P8 is an autoregulatory protein.

Two eucaryotic viruses, SV40 and adenovirus, possess autoregulatory proteins. T-antigen, the product of *gene A*, is used in a stoichiometric manner in the initiation of each round of SV40 DNA synthesis and in addition, this protein appears to control its own rate of transcription.[55]

An early transcribed gene in adenovirus type-5 specifies a 72,000 dalton protein that functions as a single stranded DNA binding protein[56] and is autogenously controlled.[57] Although in these respects the 72K protein is analogous to the gene 32 product of T_4, there is evidence that the Ad_2 DNA binding protein is involved with mRNA splicing[58] and control of mRNA translation for adenoassociated virus.[59]

V. DUAL REGULATORY PROTEINS

I have included in Table 1 five examples of regulatory proteins that have dual regulatory roles: namely, the *hut* repressor,[60] the *araC* gene product,[61] the Tn3 repressor,[62] the *lexH* gene product,[63-64] and the *tyrA* gene product.[65]

In *S. typhimurium*, histidine is catabolized to glutamate, NH_3 and formamide by a series of enzymes produced by two *hut* operons,[66] *hut MIGC* and *hut(P,R,Q) UH*. The *hutC* gene produces a repressor protein that acts on both operons. This gene product contains a binding site for urocanate, the inducer, as well as binding sites for both operators. Thus, the *hutC* gene product is autogenously controlled. This is perhaps the most clear cut example of a multifunctional regulatory protein since the independence of the two operator specific sites has been shown.[66]

In an analogous situation, the enzymes required for the catabolism of arabinose are located in the *araBAD* operon. The regulatory gene for this operon is *araC*. This operon is inducible by arabinose-*araC* gene product complex and repressible by the *araC* gene product. Lee et al.[61] propose that the *araC* gene product is autogenously controlled since discrete domains for the two overlapping promoters, Pc and P_{BAD} have been demonstrated. By analogy with the λ and *hut* repressors, the *araC* gene product would also be considered a multifunctional protein.

Thirdly, Chou et al.[62] reported on a self-regulating repressor from the Tn_3 element. Their results suggest that this regulatory protein not only controls its own synthesis, but represses translocation of the element from one carrier to another. It has not been established, however, that this repressor protein contains discrete domains.

Two laboratories[63,64] reported that the *lexA* gene is subject to autogenous control. This locus specifies a 24,000 dalton protein that serves as a repressor[63,64] of the *recA* locus, the *lexA* locus, and a locus that causes lethal filamentation when expressed. The biochemical and biophysical parameters of the *lexA* gene product as well as other regulatory molecules involved in DNA repair remain to be elucidated. It is likely, however, that this system will yield several interesting multifunctional proteins.

Lastly, the *tyrR* gene of *E. coli* produces an aporepressor protein that regulates the expression of about six operons associated with the biosynthesis and transport of aromatic amino acids. Camakaris and Pittard[65] present strong evidence that this protein is also autoregulatory. The multiple binding sites on the *tyrR* gene product include at least six for specific operator regions and three for corepressor molecules (Phe, tyr, trp), and make this protein an excellent candidate for consideration as a multifunctional regulatory protein.

VI. CONCLUSIONS

The epitome of cellular economy is exemplified with proteins that serve multifunctional roles within the cell. Since previous works have centered on multiple catalytic binding functions, the object of this chapter and book is to examine one class of proteins that have at least one regulatory cellular activity. It is premature at this point to say that all of the examples described above are multifunctional proteins in the strictest sense, and that this list is all inclusive. Nevertheless, these proteins represent a most interesting class of cellular components that require additional research on the relationship between their structure and function.

REFERENCES

1. **Jacob, F. and Monod, J.,** Genetic regulatory mechanisms in the synthesis of proteins, *J. Mol. Biol.,* 3, 318, 1961.
2. **Perlman, R., Chen, B., DeCrombrugge, B., Emmer, M., Gottesman, M., Varmus, H., and Poston, I.,** The regulation of *lac* operon transcription by cyclic adenosine 3', 5' - monophosphate, *Cold Spring Harbor Symp. Quant. Biol.,* 355, 419, 1970.
3. **Novick, A., McCoy, J. M., and Sadler, J. R.,** The noninductibility of repressor formation, *J. Mol. Biol.,* 12, 329, 1965.
4. **Maas, W. K. and McFall, E.,** Genetic aspects of metabolic control, *Annu. Rev. Microbiol.,* 18, 95, 1964.
5. **Goldberger, R. F.,** Autogenous regulation of gene expression, *Science,* 183, 810, 1974.
6. **Cove, D. J.,** Evolutionary significance of autogenous regulation, *Nature,* 251, 256, 1974.
7. **Calhoun, D. H. and Hatfield, G. W.,** Autoregulation of gene expression, *Annu. Rev. Microbiol.,* 29, 275, 1975.
8. **Savageau, M. A.,** Autogenous and classical regulation of gene expression: a general theory and experimental evidence, in *Biological Regulation and Development, Vol. 1, Gene Expression,* Goldberger, R. F., d., Plenum Press, New York, 1979, 57.
9. **Kirschner, K. and Bisswanger, H.,** Multifunctional proteins, *Annu. Rev. Biochem.,* 45, 143, 1976.
10. **Bisswanger, B. and Schminke-Ott, E., Eds.,***Multifunctional Proteins,* John Wiley & Sons, New York.
11. **Saier, M. H. and Leonard, J. E.,** The mannitol enzyme II of the bacterial phosphotransferase system: a functional chimaeric protein with receptor, transport, kinase, and regulatory activities, *Multifunctional Proteins: Catalytic/Structural and Regulatory,* Kane, J. F., Ed., CRC Press, Boca Raton, Fla., 1983, chap. 2.
12. **Menzel, R.,** The *putA* gene: two enzymatic activities and a regulatory function in a single polypeptide, *Multifunctional Proteins: Catalytic/Structural and Regulatory,* Kane, J. F., Ed., CRC Press, Boca Raton, Fla., 1983, chap. 6.

13. **Spangler, R. and Zubay, G.,** Regulation of the synthesis of the β and β′ subunits of the RNA polymerase, *Multifunctional Proteins: Catalytic/Structural and Regulatory,* Kane, J. F., Ed., CRC Press, Boca Raton, Fla., 1983, chap. 5.

14. **Putney, S. D. and Schimmel, P.,** An aminoacyl tRNA synthetase binds to a specific DNA sequence and regulates its gene transcription, *Nature,* 291, 632, 1981.

15. **Proctor, A. R. and Crawford, I. P.,** Autogenous regulation of the inducible tryptophan synthase of *Pseudomonas putida, Proc. Natl. Acad. Sci. U.S.A.,* 72, 1249, 1975.

16. **Gunsalus, I. C., Gunsalus, C. F., Chakrabarty, A. M., Sikes, S., and Crawford, I. P.,** Fine structure mapping of the tryptophan genes in *Pseudomonas putida, Genetics,* 60, 419, 1968.

17. **Proctor, A. R. and Crawford, I. P.,** Evidence for autogenous regulation of *Pseudomones putida* tryptophan synthase, *J. Bacteriol.,* 126, 548, 1976.

18. **McEntee, K.,** Protein X is the product of the *recA* gene of *Escherichia coli, Proc. Natl. Acad. Sci. U.S.A.,* 74, 5275, 1977.

19. **Roberts, J. W., Roberts, C. W., and Craig, N. L.,** *Escherichia coli recA* gene product inactivates phage λ repressor, *Proc. Natl. Acad. Sci. U.S.A.,* 75, 4714, 1978.

20. **Gudas, L. J. and Mount, D. W.,** Identification of the *recA* (tif) gene product of *Escherichia coli, Proc. Natl. Acad. Sci. U.S.A.,* 74, 5280, 1977.

21. **Shibata, T., DasGupta, C., Cunningham, R. P., and Rudding, C. M.,** Purified *Escherichia coli recA* protein catalyzes homologous pairing of superhelical DNA and single stranded fragments, *Proc. Natl. Acad. Sci. U.S.A.,* 76, 1638, 1979.

22. **McEntee, K., Weinstock, G. M., and Lehman, I. R.,** Initiation of general recombination catalyzed in vitro by the *recA* protein of *Escherichia coli, Proc. Natl. Acad. Sci. U.S.A.,* 76, 2615, 1979.

23. **Kornberg, A.,**Replication, in *DNA Synthesis,* W. H. Freeman, San Francisco, 1974, 223.

24. **Gudas, L. J. and Pardee, A. B.,** DNA synthesis inhibition and the induction of protein X in *Escherichia coli, J. Mol. Biol.,* 101, 459, 1976.

25. **Miller, H. I., Kirk, M., and Echols, H.,** SOS induction and autoregulation of the *himA* gene for site specific recombination in *Escherichia coli, Proc. Natl. Acad. Sci. U.S.A.,* 78, 6754, 1981.

26. **Sirotnak, F. M.,** High dihydrofolate reductase levels in *Diplococcus pneumoniae* after mutation in the structural gene: biochemical and immunological evidence for increased synthesis, *J. Bacteriol.,* 106, 318, 1971.

27. **Wainscott, V. J. and Kane, J. F.,** Dihydrofolate reductase in *Bacillus subtilis,* in *Microbiology — 1976,* Schlessinger, D., Ed., American Society for Microbiology, Washington, D.C., 1976, 208.

28. **Myoda, T. T., Funanage, V. L., and Young, F. E.,** Cloning and mapping of dihydrofolate reductase gene of *Bacillus subtilis, Abstr. Annu. Mtg. of Amer. Soc. Microbiol.,* 1982, 133.

29. **Myoda, T. T. and Funange, V. L.,** Gene controlling overproduction of dihydrofolate reductase and thymidylate synthetase B of *Bacillus subtilis, 4th Int. Symp. Gen. Ind. Microorganisms,* 1982, 56.

30. **Brenchley, J. E.,** Consideration of glutamine synthetase as a multifunctional protein, *Multifunctional Proteins: Catalytic/Structural and Regulatory,* Kane, J. F., Ed., CRC Press, Boca Raton, Fla., 1983, chap. 7.

31. **Hatfield, G. W. and Burns, R. O.,** Specific binding of leucyl transfer RNA to an immature form of L-threonine deaminase: its implications in repression, *Proc. Natl. Acad. Sci. U.S.A.,* 66, 1027, 1970.

32. **Kline, E. L., Brown, C. S., Coleman, W. G. Jr., and Umbarger, H. E.,** Regulation of isoleucine-valine biosynthesis in an *ilv DAC* deletion strain of *Escherichia coli* K-12, *Biochem. Biophys. Res. Commun.,* 57, 1144, 1974.

33. **Umbarger, H. E.,** Regulation of amino acid biosynthesis and regulation, *Annu. Rev. Biochem.,* 47, 533, 1978.

34. **Nargang, F. E., Subrahmanyam, C. S., and Umbarger, H. E.,** Nucleotide sequence of *ilv GEDA* operon attenuator region of *Escherichia coli, Proc. Natl. Acad. Sci. U.S.A.,* 77, 1823, 1980.

35. **Lowther, R. P. and Hatfield, G. W.,** Multivalent translational control of transcription termination at attenuator of *ilv GEDA* operon of *Escherichia coli* K 12, *Proc. Natl. Acad. Sci. U.S.A.,* 77, 1862, 1980.

36. **Bertrand, K., Korn, L., Lee, F., Platt, T., Squires, C. L., Squires, C., and Yanofsky, C.,** New features of the regulation of the tryptophan operon, *Science,* 189, 22, 1975.

37. **Ballon, A. P.,** Regulation of the *ilv l* multifunctional gene in *Sacchromyces cerevisiae, Mol. Gen. Genet.,* 142, 1, 1975.

35. **Meyers, M., Blasi, F., Bruni, C. B., Deeley, R. G., Kovach, J.S., Levinthal, M., Mullinix, K. D., Vogel, T., and Goldberger, R. F.,** Specific binding of the first enzyme for histidine biosynthesis to the DNA of the histidine operon, *Nucleic Acid Res.,* 2, 2021, 1975.

39. **Scott, J. F., Roth, J. R., and Artz, S. W.,** Regulation of histidine operon does not require *hisG* enzyme, *Proc. Natl. Acad. Sci. U.S.A.,* 72, 5021, 1975.

40. **Artz, S. W. and Broach, J. R.,** Histidine regulation in *Salmonella typhimurium:* an activator-alternator model of gene regulation, *Proc. Natl. Acad. Sci. U.S.A.,* 72, 3453, 1975.

41. **Cove, D. J. and Pateman, J. A.,** Autoregulation of the synthesis of nitrate reductase in *Aspergillus nidulans, J. Bacteriol.,* 97, 1374, 1969.

42. **Cove, D. J.,** Control of gene action in *Aspergillus nidulans, Proc. Roy. Soc. Lond. B.,* 176, 267, 1970.

43. **Kane, J. F.,** Regulation of a common amidotransferase subunit, *J. Bacteriol.,* 132, 419, 1977.

44. **Sawula, R. V. and Crawford, I. P.,** Anthranilate synthase of Acine*tobacter calcoaceticus:* separation and partial characterization of subunits, *J. Biol. Chem.,* 249, 3573, 1973.

45. **Kane, J. F. and O'Brien, H. D.,** *p* -Aminobenzoate synthase from *Bacillus subtilis:* an amidotransferase composed of non-identical subunits, *J. Bacteriol.,* 123, 1131, 1975.

46. **Holmes, W. M. and Kane, J. F.,** Anthranilate synthase from *Bacillus subtilis:* the role of a reduced subunit X in aggregate formation and amidotransferase activity, *J. Biol. Chem.,* 240, 4462, 1975.

47. **Kane, J. F. Holmes, W. M., Smiley, K. L., Jr., and Jensen, R. A.,** Rapid regulation of an anthranilate synthase aggregate by hysteresis, *J. Bacteriol.,* 113, 224, 1973.

48. **Zalkin, H.,** Anthranilate synthase: relationships between bi-functional and monofunctional enzymes, in *Multifunctional Proteins,* Bisswanger, H. and Schminke-Ott, E., Eds., Wiley-Interscience, John Wiley & Sons, New York, 1980, 123.

49. **Crawford, I. P.,** Gene fusions in the tryptophan pathway: tryptophan synthase and phosphoribosyl-anthranilate isomerase: indoleglycerol-phosphate synthase, in *Multifunctional Proteins,* Bisswanger, H. and Schwinke-Ott, E., Eds., Wiley-Interscience, John Wiley & Sons, New York, 1980, 151.

50. **Hiraga, S. and Yanofsky, C.,** Normal repression in a deletion mutant lacking almost the entire operator proximal gene of the tryptophan operon *Escherichia coli, Nature New Biol.,* 237, 47, 1972.

51. **Yates, I. and Nomura, M.,** *Escherichia coli* ribosomal proteins involved in autogenous regulation of translation, *Multifunctional Proteins: Catalytic/Structural and Regulatory,* Kane, J. F., Ed., CRC Press, Boca Raton, Fla., 1983, chap. 3.

52. **Friedman, D. I., Schauer, A. T., Baumann, M. R., Baron, L. S., and Adhya, S. L.,** Evidence that ribosomal protein S10 participates in control of transcription termination, *Proc. Natl. Acad. Sci. U.S.A.,* 78, 1115, 1981.

53. **Doherty, D. H., Gauss, P., and Gold, L.,** The single-stranded DNA binding protein of bacteriophage T4, *Multifunctional Proteins: Catalytic/Structural and Regulatory,* Kane, J. F., Ed., CRC Press, Boca Raton, Fla. 1983, chap. 3.

54. **King, J. and Casjens, S.,** Catalytic head assembling protein in virus morphogenesis, *Nature,* 251, 112, 1974.

55. **Reed, S. I., Stark, G. R., and Alwine, J. C.,** Autoregulation of simian virus 40 gene A by T antigen, *Proc. Natl. Acad. Sci. U.S.A.,* 73, 3083, 1976.

56. **Van Der Vliet, P. C., Levine, A. J., Ensinger, M. J., and Ginsberg, H. S.,** Thermolabile DNA binding proteins from cells infected with a temperature sensitive mutant of adenovirus defective in viral DNA synthesis, *J. Virol.,* 15, 348, 1975.

57. **Blanton, R. A. and Carter, T. H.,** Autoregulation of adenovirus type 5 early gene expression III. Transcription studies in isolated nuclei, *J. Virol.,* 29, 458, 1979.

58. **Myers, M. W., Laughlin, C. A., Jay, F. T., and Carter, B. J.,** Adenovirus helper function for growth of adeno-associated virus: effect of temperature-sensitive mutations in adenovirus early gene region 2, *J. Virol.,* 35, 65, 1980.

59. **Jay, F. T., Laughlin, C. A., and Carter, B. J.,** Eukaryotic translational control: abeno-associated virus protein synthesis is affected by a mutation in the adenovirus DNA-binding protein, *Proc. Natl. Acad. Sci. U.S.A.,* 75, 2927, 1981.

60. **Smith, G. R. and Magasanik, B.,** Nature and self-regulated synthesis of the repressor of the *hut* operons in *Salmonella typhimurium, Proc. Natl. Acad. Sci. U.S.A.,* 68, 1493, 1971.

61. **Lee, N. L. Gielow, W. O., and Wallace, R. G.,** Mechanism of *araC* autoregulation and the domains of two overlapping promoters, P_c and P_{BAD}, in the L-arabinose regulatory region of *Escherichia coli, Proc. Natl. Acad. Sci., U.S.A.,* 78, 752, 1981.

62. **Chou, J., Casadaban, M. J., Lemaux, P. G., and Cohen, S. W.,** Identification and characterization of a self-regulated repressor of translocation of the Tn3 element, *Proc. Natl. Acad. Sci. U.S.A.,* 76, 4020, 1979.

63. **Little, J. W. and Harper, J. E.,** Identification of the *lexA* gene product of *Escherichia coli* K12, *Proc. Natl. Acad. Sci., U.S.A.,* 76, 6147, 1979.

64. **Brent, R. and Ptashne, M.,** The *lexA* gene product represses its own promoter, *Proc. Natl. Acad. Sci. U.S.A.,* 77, 1932, 1980.

65. **Camakaris, H. and Pittard, J.,** Autoregulation of the *tyrR* gene, *J. Bacteriol.,* 150, 70, 1982.

66. **Hagen, D. C. and Magasanik, B.,** Deoxyribonucleic acid-binding studies on the *hut* repressor and mutant forms of the *hut* repressor of *Salmonella typhimurium, J. Bacteriol.,* 127, 837, 1976.

Chapter 2

THE MANNITOL ENZYME II OF THE BACTERIAL PHOSPHOTRANSFER-ASE SYSTEM: A FUNCTIONALLY CHIMAERIC PROTEIN WITH RECEPTOR, TRANSPORT, KINASE, AND REGULATORY ACTIVITIES

Milton H. Saier, Jr. and John E. Leonard

TABLE OF CONTENTS

I. INTRODUCTION

Recent studies have revealed that many enzymes catalyze more than a single chemical reaction and that their activities may be subject to allosteric regulation by ligands or proteins which are not structurally related to the substrates or products of the enzyme catalyzed reactions. The allosteric effectors bind to sites on the protein which are topologically distinct from the active sites involved in catalysis.[1] Additionally, a few of these proteins in bacteria function in the regulation of their own syntheses either at the transcriptional or the translational level. Several examples of such proteins are discussed in this volume. In general, these enzymes are cytoplasmic constituents which can freely diffuse to the bacterial chromosome or to the appropriate messenger RNA molecules where they exert their regulatory roles.

There is evidence that a few membrane-associated proteins mediating the transmembrane transport of sugars may also function in transcriptional regulation. Thus, the product of the *malK* gene in *E. coli*,[2] and the Enzyme III[lac] of the lactose phosphotransferase system of *Staphylococcus aureus*,[3] may both function directly in transcriptional regulation of their respective regulons.[4] Integral transmembrane proteins may also control the rates of DNA transcription by mechanisms which depend on their interactions with cytoplasmic transcriptional repressors or activators.[5] The latter proteins presumably bind to the regulatory regions of the target operons as well as to the transmembrane proteins, and an equilibrium situation, determining the amount of the regulatory protein associated with the nucleic acid, may control the rate of mRNA synthesis.[4,5]

In this chapter we shall discuss our recent findings concerned with the catalytic and regulatory properties of the mannitol Enzyme II of the *E. coli* phosphotransferase system (PTS). Our success in solubilizing this enzyme and obtaining it in pure form,[6] in cloning the mannitol *mtl* operon,[7] and in developing a simple, rapid, positive selection procedure for the isolation of mutants altered for the Enzyme II[Mtl] structural gene *mtlA*[8] render the mannitol Enzyme II presently the best characterized, and also the most amenable to future investigation, of the integral PTS group translocating enzymes.

II. PHYSIOLOGICAL FUNCTIONS OF MANNITOL ENZYME II IN *E. coli*

Figure 1 shows the pathway for the initiation of D-mannitol catabolism in *E. coli*. The sugar is transported across the membrane and concomitantly phosphorylated by a PTS-mediated mechanism. In this process the phosphoryl group of phosphoenolpyruvate is transferred sequentially from phosphoenolpyruvate to Enzyme I and HPr, the two energy coupling proteins of the phosphotransferase system. Phospho-HPr then binds to the cytoplasmic surface of the Enzyme II,[Mtl] and free mannitol, in the extracellular medium, approaches the sugar binding site on the outer face of the enzyme. Group translocation of the sugar through the membrane corresponds to the simultaneous transport and phosphorylation of the substrate, with the release of D-mannitol-1-phosphate in the cytoplasm. The byproduct of this reaction is pyruvate. Cytoplasmic mannitol-1-phosphate is then oxidized to fructose-6-phosphate in a process catalyzed by mannitol-1-phosphate dehydrogenase in which NAD^+ serves as the electron acceptor. While the general energy coupling proteins of the PTS, Enzyme I, and HPr, are coded for by the *ptsI* and *ptsH* genes, respectively, which comprise the *pts* operon,[9,10] the Enzyme II[Mtl] and the mannitol-1-phosphate dehydrogenase are coded for by the *mtlA* and *mtlD* genes, respectively, which comprise the *mtl* operon.[11,12,13] Substantial differences between the protein constituents of the PTS in the two principal organisms under study, *E. coli* and *S. typhimurium,* have not been revealed by available investigations.

The mannitol Enzyme II apparently functions in the bacterial cell in multiple capacities.

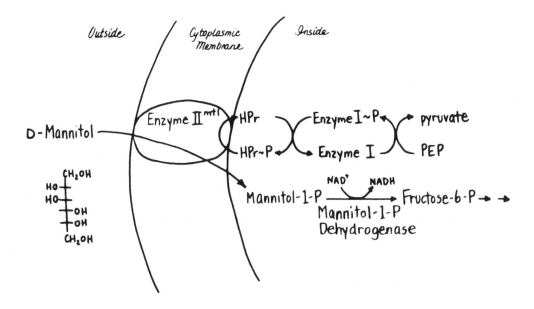

FIGURE 1. Pathway of D-mannitol utilization in *E. coli* and *S. typhimurium*.

The different functions are summarized in Table 1. Adler and his collaborators[14,15] as well as Melton and Hartman[16] have provided evidence that the Enzymes II of the PTS function as receptors for chemotactic processes which occur in response to gradients of the substrate sugars of the PTS. Thus, the mannitol chemoreceptor is apparently the Enzyme II[Mtl]. The Enzyme II also catalyzes both unidirectional and bidirectional exchange translocation of its sugar substrate (Table 1 and References 5 and 17). These vectorial processes are coupled respectively to the phosphoenolpyruvate-dependent and mannitol-1-phosphate-dependent phosphorylation of mannitol. Thus, unidirectional transport is driven by phospho-HPr (or ultimately by phosphoenolpyruvate) while bidirectional exchange transport is driven by mannitol-1-phosphate.[5]

In addition to the catalytic functions discussed above, the Enzyme II[Mtl] functions indirectly in a number of regulatory processes. It apparently can promote the transcriptional induction of the *pts* operon in a process dependent on extracellular mannitol, and it mediates the regulation of the activities of adenylate cyclase and a number of nonPTS permeases.[5] In each of these processes, regulation is presumed to result from the presence of a protein which can itself be phosphorylated at the expense of phosphoenolpyruvate. The mannitol Enzyme II may effect dephosphorylation of this regulatory protein.[5]

Recently, we have obtained preliminary evidence for an additional regulatory function of this enzyme, involving autoinduction of the *mtl* operon. In this chapter we shall concentrate first on some of the interesting transport and phosphorylation functions of the Enzyme II[Mtl], and secondly on the possible involvement of the protein in transcriptional regulation. The reader is referred to recent reviews for comprehensive discussions of less current aspects of Enzyme II[Mtl] function.[5,18,19]

III. ALTERNATIVE DISPOSITIONS OF ENZYME II[Mtl] IN MEMBRANE VESICLES OF *E. coli*

As noted above, the Enzyme II[Mtl] catalyzes two distinct group translocation processes, unidirectional sugar uptake driven by phospho-HPr, and bidirectional exchange group trans-

Table 1

**FUNCTIONS OF THE MANNITOL ENZYME II OF THE BACTERIAL
PHOSPHOTRANSFERASE SYSTEM**

    I.   Catalytic activities
        A.   Mannitol chemoreceptor
        B.   Mannitol permease
            1.   Unidirectional group translocation
            2.   Bidirectional group translocation
        C.   Mannitol kinase
            1.   Phosphoenolpyruvate as phosphoryl donor
            2.   Mannitol 1-phosphate as phosphoryl donor
    II.   Regulatory functions (direct or indirect)
        A.   Induction of *pts* operon expression
        B.   Control of adenylate cyclase and non-PTS permease activities
        C.   Autoinduction of *mtl* operon expression

location as illustrated in Figure 2. In the latter process an extracellular molecule of mannitol is transported into the cell and simultaneously phosphorylated while the sugar moiety of a cytoplasmic mannitol-1-phosphate molecule is transported out. The phosphoryl moiety of the outgoing sugar is thus transferred to the incoming sugar. On the cytoplasmic face of the Enzyme II there are apparently separate binding sites for phospho-HPr and sugar phosphate. An essential sulfhydryl group is localized to the cytoplasmic surface. On the external face of this transmembrane enzyme is the sugar binding site.[20,21] It is also possible that the bidirectional exchange process requires a more aggregated state of the enzyme than that required to catalyze unidirectional transport (see below).

In a series of recent studies, it was found in membrane vesicles of *E. coli* that the Enzyme II[Mtl] can apparently catalyze nonvectorial as well as vectorial phosphorylation of radioactive mannitol both by the phosphoenolpyruvate-dependent and by the mannitol-1-phosphate-dependent reactions (Table 2 and Reference 22). Of particular interest was the fact that the membrane impermeable reagent, *p*-chloromercuriphenyl sulfonate (pCMPS)[23] completely abolished the nonvectorial reaction without inhibiting the vectorial reaction. Further, studies showed that the enzyme population catalyzing the nonvectorial reaction possessed an extravesicular sugar phosphate binding site although the enzyme population catalyzing the vectorial reaction did not.[22]

These results were obtained employing osmotically shocked membrane vesicles of *E. coli*. When the disposition of the Enzymes II was examined in intact cells of *E. coli*, *Salmonella typhimurium*, *Bacillus subtilis*, and *Staphylococcus aureus* it was found that only a single enzyme orientation could be demonstrated, that in which the essential sulfhydryl group and the sugar phosphate binding site were exposed to the cytoplasm. Thus, in contrast to the suggestion made in Reference 22, the nonvectorial reaction is an artifact of vesicle preparation. The nature of the randomization process which allows the cytoplasmic surface of the Enzymes II to become exposed to the extravesicular medium during osmotic shock is not understood.

IV. EVIDENCE FOR FUNCTIONAL AGGREGATION OF PURIFIED ENZYME II[Mtl] IN LUBROL MICELLES

In order to understand the catalytic and physicochemical properties of the mannitol Enzyme II, the protein was solubilized from the membrane with deoxycholate in the presence of 0.2 *M* salt and purified to homogeneity employing a variety of techniques including hydrophobic chromatography and hydrophobic ion exchange chromatography.[6] A single protein band was

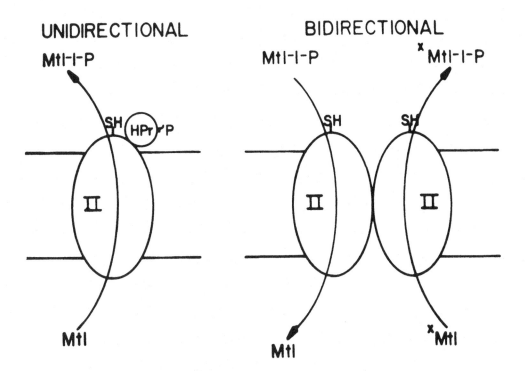

FIGURE 2. Schematic depiction of the two vectorial reactions catalyzed by the mannitol Enzyme II. The hypothetical subunit dependencies are discussed in the text.

Table 2
SELECTIVE INHIBITION OF NON-VECTORIAL
TRANSPHOSPHORYLATION RELATIVE TO
THE VECTORIAL PROCESS, AS CATALYZED
BY THE MANNITOL ENZYME II IN
MEMBRANE VESICLES OF *E. coli* **STRAIN ML308**

Sugar (10 μ M)	p-CMPS (0.1 m M)	Rate of transphosphorylation (nmol/min per mg protein)	
		Vectorial	**Nonvectorial**
Mannitol	−	0.43	0.86
Mannitol	+	0.44	0

(Data taken from Saier, M. H., Jr. and Schmidt, M. R., *J. Bacteriol.*, 145, 391, 1981. With permission.)

observed by polyacrylamide gel electrophoresis either in the presence or absence of sodium dodecylsulfate. Eight different preparations of the protein had isoelectric points between 6.2 and 7.0 (Figure 3). Studies with the purified protein suggested that it was a single polypeptide chain with a molecular weight of about 60,000 daltons. As expected for a large integral membrane protein, the amino acid composition revealed a moderate degree of hydrophobicity (40 to 45%).[47] The purified polypeptide catalyzed both the mannitol-1-phosphate-dependent transphosphorylation reaction and the phosphoenolpyruvate-dependent phosphorylation of mannitol at the same *relative* rates as in the native membrane, but the specific activities of the two reactions were increased about 200-fold relative to the broken cell preparation. While

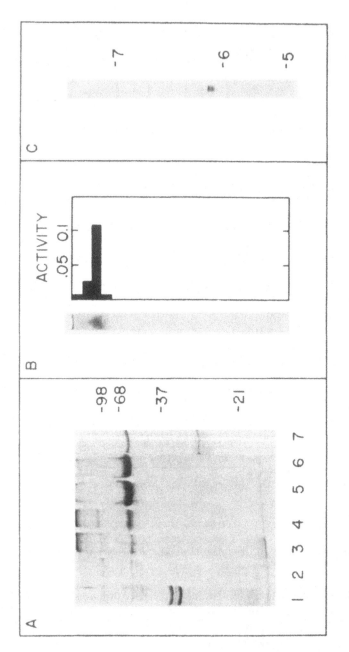

FIGURE 3.   Gel electrophoretic analyses of the enzyme II^Mtl (A) Gel analyses of the protein preparations during purification. (B) Conventional gel electrophoresis of the active enzyme in detergent solution. (C) Isoelectric focussing of the purified enzyme. (From Jacobson, G. R., Lee, C. A., and Saier, M. H., Jr., *J. Biol. Chem.*, 254, 249, 1979. With permission.) Conditions were as described therein.

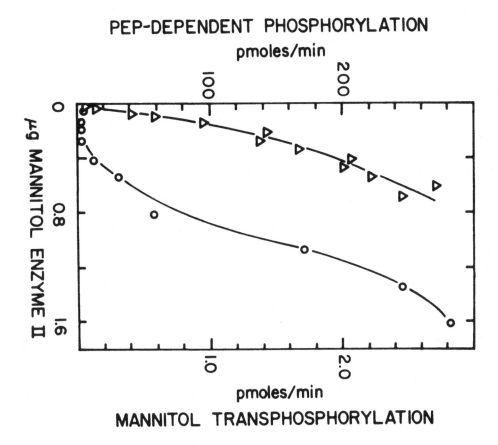

PEP-DEPENDENT PHOSPHORYLATION
pmoles/min

MANNITOL TRANSPHOSPHORYLATION
pmoles/min

FIGURE 4. The dependencies of the rates of the phosphoenolpyruvate-dependent (Δ-Δ) and mannitol-1-phosphate-dependent (o-o) mannitol phosphorylation reactions on the concentration of mannitol Enzyme II. Both phosphorylation reactions were catalyzed by purified mannitol Enzyme II at a constant nonionic detergent (Lubrol PX) concentration of 0.5%. In each case less than 10% of the available radiolabeled substrate was consumed during the course of the reaction. The general proteins of the PTS, Enzyme I and HPr, required for the PEP-dependent phosphorylation of mannitol, were purified as described by Kundig and Roseman[45] and Anderson et al[46] and supplied to the reaction mixture in excess of the amounts required. The PEP-dependent assays were conducted essentially as described previously.[24,45] The mannitol-1-phosphate reaction was assayed essentially as described previously[6] except that the final concentrations of mannitol and mannitol-1-phosphate were 0.5 μM and 1 mM, respectively.

the activity of the crude membrane bound enzyme or the crude deoxycholate extract was stimulated by addition of the nonionic detergent, Lubrol, the activity of the purified enzyme in Lubrol was stimulated as much as three-fold by addition of purified phospholipids. Of the phospholipids tested, phosphatidylglycerol was most stimulatory followed by phosphatidylethanolamine and phosphatidylcholine.[48]

Evidence for functional association of protomeric species of the Enzyme II was obtained by studying the two activities of the purified enzyme as a function of enzyme concentration at a constant concentration of Lubrol micelles (Figure 4).[49] As revealed by the results depicted in the figure, an activity vs. enzyme concentration plot gave a hyperbolic curve for the phosphoenolpyruvate-dependent reaction. By contrast, a sigmoidal curve was observed for the transphosphorylation reaction regardless of the pH of the medium and under all conditions examined. Although other interpretations can be entertained, these results can be explained by a self-association type process if it is assumed that the associated form of the enzyme catalyzes the transphosphorylation reaction more rapidly than the disaggregated form. Figure

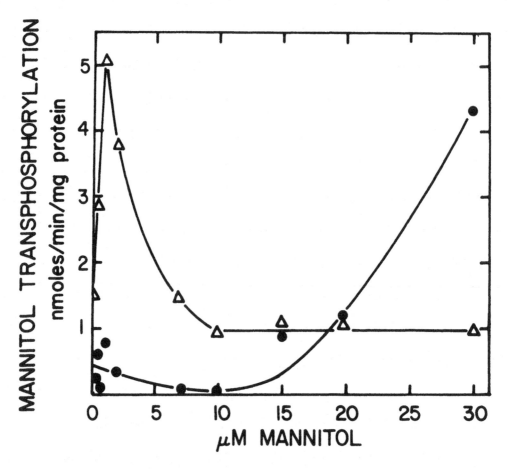

FIGURE 5.   Effect of Enzyme II^{Mtl} concentration on transphosphorylation activity as a function of [^{14}C] mannitol concentration. The rate of the mannitol transphosphorylation reaction was studied as a function of the mannitol concentration at two different mannitol Enzyme II concentrations. The mannitol Enzyme II used in these assays was purified as described previously,[6] and two different but constant levels of enzyme were used in the assay. The low Enzyme II^{Mtl} concentration was 0.34 μg/mℓ (●-●) and the high enzyme concentration (Δ-Δ) was 4.0 μg/mℓ. The nonionic detergent (Lubrol PX) concentration (0.5%) was held constant throughout the assays. The concentration of mannitol-1-phosphate was held constant at 1 mM.

5 reveals an additional interesting feature of the association process. At low enzyme concentration, virtually no transphosphorylation activity was observed for the enzyme below a substrate concentration of 15 μM mannitol, and no substrate inhibition occurred at mannitol concentrations in excess of 30 μM when the conditions reported in the figure caption were employed. By contrast, when the enzyme concentration was increased 10-fold, maximal activity was observed at about 1 μM sugar, and strong substrate inhibition resulted when the mannitol concentration was increased above this value (Figure 5). Further studies revealed that at higher enzyme concentration the enzyme appeared to exhibit higher affinity for mannitol than the dissociated form when the phosphoryl donor was phospho-HPr (unpublished results). These results suggest that if self-association is responsible for the reported observations, it has several effects on catalytic function of the Enzyme II^{Mtl}: (1) it specifically facilitates catalysis of the mannitol-1-phosphate:mannitol transphosphorylation reaction; (2) it enhances the affinity of the enzyme for mannitol as the sugar substrate; and (3) it promotes and is perhaps required for substrate inhibition. It is possible that the phenomenon of substrate inhibition of transphosphorylation, a general characteristic of this type of reaction,[5] is only

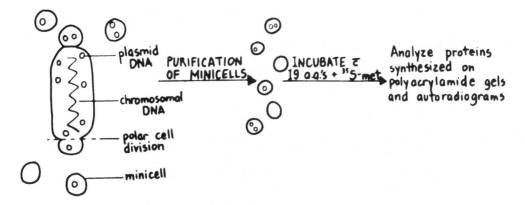

A <u>minA, minB</u> strain (MV1009) has aberrant cell division and produces minicells. Minicells contain no chromosomal DNA, only plasmid DNA.

FIGURE 6.   Schematic depiction of the use of minicells to study proteins encoded by the hybrid *mtl* plasmid. The *minA minB* strain of *E. coli* employed (strain MV 1009) possesses abberant cell division which gives rise to minicells. Minicells contain no chromosomal DNA but do contain plasmid DNA.

observed when the protomers of the enzyme are associated. If so, an allosteric type mechanism rather than a simple competitive mechanism may be operative.

V. EXPRESSION OF CLONED *mtl* OPERON IN *E. coli* MINI-CELLS

In order to gain an understanding of the biosynthetic processes and regulatory events which control expression of the mannitol operon and to unequivocally identify the *mtl* gene products, the mannitol operon was cloned, and its expression was studied in mini-cells derived from a *minA minB* double mutant strain of *E. coli* (strain MV1009).[7] This strain exhibits aberrant cell division such that it produces "minicells" which contain plasmid DNA, but no chromosomal DNA (Figure 6). After separation of the mini-cells from the parental cells, the former are capable of directing the synthesis of proteins encoded by plasmid DNA exclusively. Analysis of these proteins is possible after labeling them with ^{35}S-methionine or another radioactive amino acid and electrophoretically separating the radiolabeled proteins in acrylamide gels containing sodium dodecylsulfate. The results obtained with one plasmid, pLC 15-48, encoding the mannitol operon, are reproduced in Figure 7. In the absence of cyclic AMP and inducer (mannitol) no proteins were synthesized in the minicells in appreciable amounts. Addition of both cyclic AMP and mannitol was required to promote expression of the mannitol operon,[7,12,13] and two major proteins were synthesized in response to these two regulatory agents. One was a soluble protein with a molecular weight of about 40,000 daltons; the other was an integral membrane protein of 60,000 daltons. Because the size of the mannitol-1-phosphate dehydrogenase is about 40,000 daltons[47] we assume the cytoplasmic protein to be this enzyme. In order to establish that the radioactive protein in the envelope fraction was the Enzyme II[Mtl], the envelope was solubilized and the radiolabeled protein was shown to be precipitated quantitatively by anti-mannitol Enzyme II antibody. Preimmune antibody was ineffective in precipitating the radioactive protein. It can therefore be concluded that the mannitol operon encodes a single integral membrane protein which is identical to the Enzyme II[Mtl]. Since the mannitol chemoreceptor, permease and phosphoenolpyruvate-dependent kinase are all known to be inducible by mannitol[19] and

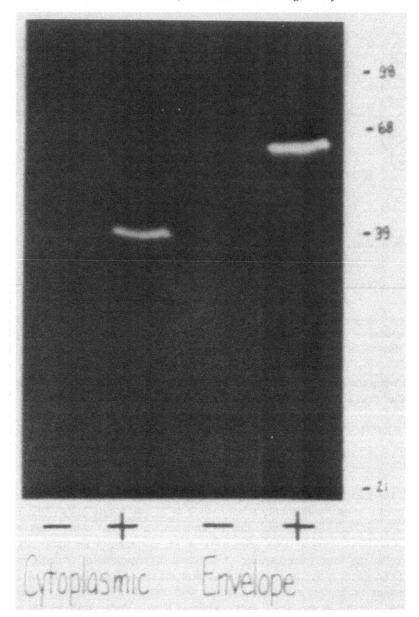

FIGURE 7. Characterization of the proteins encoded by plasmid pLC15-48 in minicells. Minicells were incubated with (+) or without (−) mannitol and cyclic AMP. Subsequently the cytoplasmic and envelope fractions were separated by centrifugation and analyzed by polyacrylamide gel electrophoresis in the presence of sodium dodecyl sulfate. Procedures were as described in Lee, C. A., Jacobson, G. R., and Saier, M. H., Jr., *Proc. Natl. Acad. Sci.*, 78, 7336, 1981.

are membrane associated, we conclude from this experiment that all three activities are attributable to the mannitol Enzyme II protein.

VI. EVOLUTIONARY RELATIONSHIPS BETWEEN PROTEINS OF THE PHOSPHOTRANSFERASE SYSTEM

In 1977 we proposed a scheme for the evolution of genes coding for proteins of the *E. coli* and *S. typhimurium* PTS.[26] This scheme, reproduced in Figure 8, is based upon results

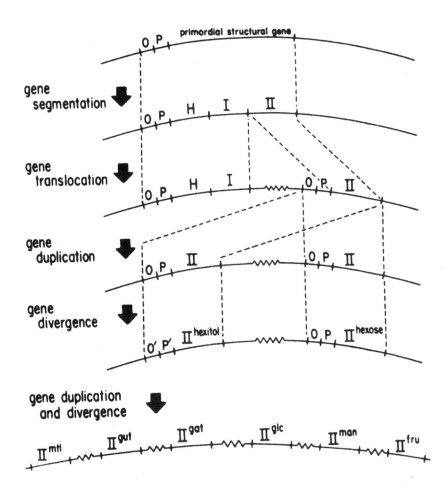

FIGURE 8. Proposed scheme for the evolution of the genetic apparatus encoding protein constituents of the complex PTS found in *E. coli* or *S. typhimurium*. The abbreviations are *mtl*, mannitol; *gut*, glucitol; *gat*, galactitol; *glc*, glucose; *man*, mannose; *fru*, fructose. The scheme was proposed previously.[24]

obtained when phosphotransferase systems were characterized from a number of evolutionarily divergent bacterial genera including *Rhodospirillum, Rhodopseudomonas, Spirochaeta, Megasphera,* and *Salmonella.*[5,26] It is assumed that the genetic precursor of the PTS was a single cistron coding for a kinase-type protein which possibly originated as a soluble constituent. Mutations which caused substitution of hydrophobic amino acid residues for hydrophilic residues within a region of the product polypeptide chain may have brought about association of the protein with the cytoplasmic membrane of the primordial bacterium. Introduction of nonsense mutations in the chain, possibly following duplication of parts of the gene, may then have given rise to distinct soluble and membrane associated constituents still under the control of a single operator-promotor region. Such a situation probably still prevails with the phosphotransferase systems found in *Rhodospirillum,*[27] *Rhodopseudomonas,*[27] and *Spirochaeta aurantia.*[17,28] Separation of the primordial Enzyme II gene from the genes coding for the soluble energy coupling proteins of the system must have occurred relatively early in evolutionary history. The former gene must have then duplicated and diverged such that evolving genes coding for the Enzymes II of the PTS may have exhibited specificities for hexitols, for aldohexoses, and for fructose. Finally, additional duplications and further diversion must have given rise to the mannitol, glucitol, and galactitol Enzyme

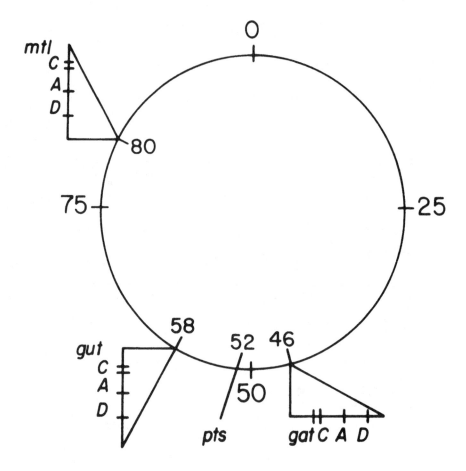

FIGURE 9.   Map of the *E. coli* chromosome showing the hexitol operons and their presumed gene orders.

II genes, all derived from the primordial hexitol gene. The primordial hexose gene presumably also underwent duplication to yield the mannose, glucose, N-acetylglucosamine, and β-glucoside Enzyme II complexes. If this hypothesis were correct then one would expect that some of the Enzyme II operons which diverged most recently in evolutionary history would retain some common catalytic, structural and regulatory features. In fact, overlapping substrate specificities of the glucose, mannose, N-acetylglucosamine, and β-glucoside Enzymes II have been reported.[20,21,29-31] Moreover, expression of the mannose and glucose Enzyme II genes exhibit common regulatory properties.[32]

Still more convincing are the data of Lengeler[12,13] which show that the three operons encoding the hexitol catabolic enzyme systems in *E. coli* exhibit similar gene orders: the mannitol operon consists of a *cis* dominant regulatory region *(mtlC)* followed by the two known structural genes, *mtlA* and *mtlD*, which respectively code for the mannitol Enzyme II and mannitol-1-phosphate dehydrogenase. The same three genes have been tentatively identified within the glucitol and galactitol operons (Figure 9), and fine structure mapping suggests that the gene order is the same. In view of the suggestion that the present day *E. coli* chromosome evolved as a result of two complete duplications of a primordial chromosome one-quarter of its present size,[33] it is interesting that the hexitol catabolic operons are found within three of the four quadrants of the chromosome (Figure 9). It is worth noting that the three hexitol Enzymes II exhibit overlapping substrate specificites which include a variety of polyols,[12,13] as well as fructose.[34] In view of the probable evolutionary relatedness

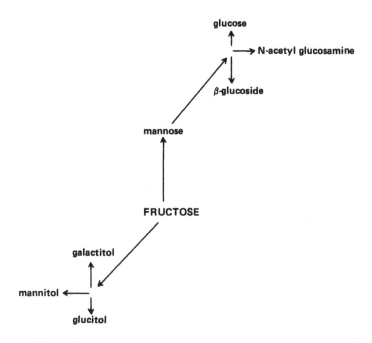

FIGURE 10.   Proposed evolutionary relatedness of enzymes II of the *E. coli*
PTS. The scheme indicates directionality in the evolutionary process as discussed
in the text.

of the hexitol operons, it would not be at all surprising if the regulatory mechanisms
controlling their expression exhibited common features. Regulatory proteins for the hexitol
operons might exhibit common structural features and might even substitute for one another
under appropriate conditions. The results discussed below allow us to entertain these
possibilities.

The possible relatedness of different Enzymes II of the PTS was investigated by using
antibodies directed against homogeneous Enzyme II.^{Mtl} The inhibitory effects of low antibody
concentrations on the activities of the different Enzymes II were examined. The results were
as follows:

$$II^{Mtl} > II^{Gut} > II^{Fru} > II^{Man} > II^{Glc} = II^{Nag}$$

These results and other considerations led to a proposal of the evolutionary scheme shown
in Figure 10. In this scheme we suggest that the primordial Enzyme II gene (Figure 8) may
have encoded a fructose specific enzyme. Several independent considerations lead to this
suggestion:

1.   Anaerobic glycolysis was undoubtedly the first sugar degradative pathway to evolve,
     and fructose is the only hexose which feeds directly into the glycolytic scheme without
     epimerization or isomerization. Thus, fewer enzymes are required for its metabolism
     than for other sugars found in nature.

2.   A large number of Gram-negative bacterial genera which lack a general PTS do
     metabolize fructose via a pathway which is initiated by phosphoenolpyruvate-dependent
     phosphotransferase systems. Included among these genera are *Rhodospirillum*,[27] *Rho-
     dopseudomonas*,[27] *Thiocapsa*,[35] *Alcaligenes*,[36] *Pseudomonas*,[37,38] *Fusobacterium*,[39] and
     others. Those bacterial species which have been studied apparently possess HPr-
     independent phosphorylation systems containing only two known proteins, one integral
     membrane protein complex, and one peripheral membrane protein.[27,51]

3.   The fructose PTS in *E. coli* and *S. typhimurium* is the only one in these organisms which can function in the absence of HPr.[6,7,52] Thus, the simpler fructose specific phosphotransferase systems found in the Gram-negative genera noted above apparently may be retained in enteric bacteria which possess a complex PTS.

Duplication and divergence of a primordial Enzyme II[Fru] gene may have given rise to a hexitol Enzyme II gene and a general hexose Enzyme II gene in addition to the fructose Enzyme II gene. Both would initially exhibit broad specificities, the former for a variety of polyols, the latter for a number of hexoses. Thus, the evolving hexose enzyme would have been analogous to the present day mannose Enzyme II of *E. coli* and *S. typhimurium* (Figure 10).[21] Each of these two ancestral genes must have then duplicated and diverged further to yield the individual hexitol and hexose Enzyme II genes coding for enzymes with restricted specificity as indicated in Figure 10. As the most recent duplications presumably involved the complete operons, one can anticipate similar or overlapping modes of regulation.

VII. POSSIBLE INVOLVEMENT OF ENZYME II[Mtl] IN REGULATING MANNITOL OPERON TRANSCRIPTION

Several publications have suggested that a link might exist between mannitol and glucitol utilization in enteric bacteria. Although the catabolic enzyme systems which initiate the degradation of these two hexitols are encoded by distinct genes within distinct operons (Figure 9), Berkowitz first reported that mutants of *S. typhimurium* which were isolated on the basis of defective mannitol utilization often fermented glucitol poorly relative to the parental strain.[11]

Several years ago Englesberg described a procedure for the isolation of glucose-methyl α-glucoside permease negative mutants in *Salmonella typhimurium*.[40,41] Parental mutant strains which lack the enzyme, phosphoenolpyruvate carboxylase, due to a mutation in the *ppc* gene, cannot synthesize Krebs cycle intermediates from sugars which are metabolized via glycolysis. While *ppc* mutants can ordinarily grow if an exogenous source of citrate is available, the mutants cannot grow in minimal salts medium supplemented with citrate and glucose.[40,41] The reason for glucose induced growth stasis is that glucose supresses synthesis of the citrate permease, thereby preventing uptake of citrate into the cells. On such media, mutants capable of growth arise which lack the glucose permease, and these mutants are defective for the glucose Enzyme II of the PTS.[8] Moreover, glucose could be replaced by fructose or mannitol, as these sugars also repressed the synthesis of the citrate permease.[8] Mutants isolated for their ability to grow on citrate plus fructose or citrate plus mannitol were frequently defective for the fructose or mannitol Enzyme II, respectively, as expected.

In subsequent studies[42] 60 *mtlA* mutants, defectie for the mannitol Enzyme II, were isolated by this procedure, and they were characterized by assays which measured the various activities catalyzed by this enzyme. The mutants fell into six classes as summarized in Table 3.[42] Class I mutants lacked all activities associated with the Enzyme II[Mtl] (mannitol chemotaxis, transport, PEP-dependent mannitol phosphorylation, and mannitol-1-phosphate-dependent transphosphorylation). These mutants presumably included nonsense and deletion mutants and may therefore lack the Enzyme II[Mtl] protein altogether. Class II mutants lacked each of the four activities assayed with the exception of transphosphorylation which was near the wild type level. The sugar and sugar phosphate binding sites of the Enzyme II had to be intact in these mutants. Class III and IV mutants showed depressed levels of all activities with the exception of chemotaxis. While Class III mutants showed elevated chemotactic responses to mannitol, Class IV mutants showed no detectable response.[42] In these mutants the chemotactic function of the Enzyme II was dissected from the other activities. Class V mutants showed an elevation of all activities except for phosphoenolpyruvate-

Table 3
CLASSES OF ENZYME II^Mtl MUTANTS (*mtlA*)

Class	Transport	Chemotaxis	PEP-dependent phosphorylation	Mannitol-1-P -dependent phosphorylation
Parent	+	+	+	+
I	−	−	−	−
II	−	−	−	+
III	±	+ +	±	±
IV	±	−	±	±
V	+ +	+ +	±	+ +
VI	±	±	±	±

(From Leonard, J. E. and Saier, M. H., Jr., *J. Bacteriol.*, 145, 1106, 1981. With permission.)

Table 4
PROPERTIES OF TWO *mtlA* MUTANT CLASSES OF *SALMONELLA TYPHIMURIUM*

Property	LT-2	*S. typhimurium* Strain Mutant class I	Mutant class II
Mannitol			
Fermentation	+	−	−
Transport	+	−	−
Chemotaxis	+	−	−
PEP-dependent phosphorylation	+	−	−
Mannitol-1-P-dependent phosphorylation	+	−	+
Mannitol-1-P dehydrogenase	Inducible	Noninducible	Constitutive

Note: The two classes shown are Classes I and II from Table 3.[42] Assay and growth conditions were described in Table 5.

dependent phosphorylation which was substantially depressed. Finally, in Class VI mutants, all activities of the Enzyme II were depressed. This class is the trivial class of "leaky" mutants where the genetic defect did not have a selective effect on any one activity of the enzyme.

When the levels of the mannitol-1-phosphate dehydrogenase were examined in these various classes of mutants, a surprising result was obtained. While the parental strain was inducible for the dehydrogenase to the extent of 20-fold, little or no induction was observed for Class I mutants (Table 4). By contrast, Class II mutants exhibited high constitutive activities of the dehydrogenase, roughly comparable to those observed with the fully induced parent. Classes III to VI showed partial induction.

Data quantitating these qualitative observations are recorded in Table 5. The noninducibility of the mannitol-1-phosphate dehydrogenase in two representative Class I mutants is contrasted with the constitutivity of two Class II mutants. Of even greater surprise was the observation that the levels of glucitol-6-phosphate dehydrogenase were affected by the

Table 5

INDUCTION OF MANNITOL-P DEHYDROGENASE IN CLASS I AND CLASS II
***mtlA* MUTANTS**

Induction of mannitol-phosphate dehydrogenase in class I and class II *mtlA* mutants of *Salmonella typhimurium*. The mutants were isolated from Strain SB2956 as described previously.[42] Overnight cultures in L broth were used to inoculate L broth medium containing D-mannitol at a final concentration of 0.4% (w/v); uninduced cultures were grown in medium LB alone. All cultures were harvested in mid-log phase growth and washed three times by successive centrifugation and resuspension in medium 63 containing no carbon source; the final resuspension was in 4 mℓ of the same. The washed cells were then ruptured in the presence of 1 mM dithiothreitol by passage through a French press at 15,000 lb/in². Whole cells were removed by low speed centrifugation, and the cell membrane fragments were subsequently separated from the soluble proteins by centrifugation at 100,000 × g for 90 min at 4°C. The mannitol-1-phosphate dehydrogenase assay solutions contained in a final volume of 1 mℓ: 3-15 μg protein, 60 μℓ of 25 mM β-NAD$^+$, 5 μℓ of 0.2 M mannitol-1-phosphate, and 930-934 μℓ of 0.1 M Tris-HCl buffer, pH 8.9 (23°). The assays were followed by observing the reduction of β-NAD$^+$ at 340 nm.

Class	Strain	Mannitol-P dehydrogenase (μmoles/min/mg, protein)	
		− Inducer	$^+$Inducer
	SB2956	0.2	5.2
I	LJ407	0.2	0.5
I	LJ409	0.1	0.1
II	LJ414	4.8	5.1
II	LJ415	5.8	7.3

mannitol Enzyme II mutations in qualitatively similar fashion (data not shown). While the Class I mutants showed slow induction of the glucitol-6-phosphate dehydrogenase, the Class II mutants synthesized the enzyme semiconstitutively under the conditions employed.

Table 6 records the results of similar assays carried out with deletion mutants lacking the *pts* operon which codes for HPr and Enzyme I of the PTS. The mannitol-p dehydrogenases was synthesized constitutively in these strains.

One additional interesting feature of mannitol operon regulation has come to light. Yashphe and Kaplan[43] characterized mannitol specific pseudorevertants of mutant strains of *E. coli* which lacked either the cyclic AMP receptor protein (*crp* mutants) or adenylate cyclase (*cya* mutants). Some of these strains synthesized the mannitol-1-phosphate dehydrogenase constitutively, suggesting that the operator and promoter of the mannitol operon overlap functionally and possibly structurally. Recently, similar mutations have been isolated on the plasmid pLC 15-48.[53] Some of the mutations appear to map within the *mtlA* gene, further substantiating the conclusion that the mannitol Enzyme II plays a role in transcriptional regulation of the operon.[53] The major observations and conclusions described above are summarized in Table 7.

Figure 11 shows a highly schematic and speculative model to explain the possible involvement of the Enzyme II^{Mtl} in transcriptional regulation of the mannitol operon. It is suggested that in the wild type bacterium, the enzyme can exist in at least two conformations: one is phosphorylated (or has phospho-HPr bound to the cytoplasmic surface) and is inactive as a transcriptional activator. This conformation of the protein is analogous to complete loss of function (Class I *mtlA* mutants[42]). The other conformation is induced when mannitol binds to the active site, and phosphate is drained off of the enzyme. This latter conformation is presumed to function as a transcriptional activator and is the conformation in which the enzyme is locked in Class II *mtlA* mutants and deletion *pts* mutants. It should be pointed out that the mechanism of transcriptional regulation is unknown at this time. The Enzyme II^{Mtl} might not interact directly with the DNA, but might instead control the cytoplasmic

Table 6
EXPRESSION OF *mtl* OPERON IN
pts MUTANTS OF *S.*
TYPHIMURIUM[a]

Strain	Mannitol-P dehydrogenase (μmol/min/mg protein)	
	− Inducer	⁺Inducer
LT2	0.2	4.0
Δ *ptsHI41*	4.5	4.0
Δ *ptsHIcrrA49*	7.7	7.3

Note: Expression of the *mtlD* gene in strains of
S. typhimurium which were deleted from
the *pts* operon. Growth and assay conditions were described in Table 5.

[a] Growth and assay conditions were as described in Table 4.

Table 7
TRANSCRIPTIONAL REGULATION OF *mtl* OPERON

Observations
1. *mtlA* Mutations → non-inducible, semi-inducible, or constitutive expression
2. *ptsH*, *ptsI* and *ptsHI* Mutations → semi-constitutive or constitutive expression
3. *mtl*-Specific pseudorevertants of *crp* or *cya* mutants → inducible or constitutive expression

Tentative Conclusions
1. Enzyme II^Mtl regulates *mtl* operon expression by an activator-type mechanism
2. Interaction of phospho-HPr with EII^mtl or phosphorylation of EII^mtl neutralizes the activation
3. The operator and promoter sites overlap

concentration of an inducer or a soluble regulatory protein which does bind to the operator-promoter region.[5] Relevant to this possibility is a recent report by Csonka and Clark[44] which suggests that a negative regulatory protein (repressor), distinct from the Enzymes II, is encoded by the *gutR* gene, adjacent to the glucitol operon in *S. typhimurium*.

VIII. CONCLUSIONS

Our recent efforts to elucidate the mechanisms of Enzyme II mediated functions have resulted in the isolation of homogeneous Enzyme II^Mtl and in the cloning of mannitol operon DNA. A restriction map of the plasmid pLC 15-48 is now available,[54] and the complete DNA sequence of the operon should be available in the foreseeable future. These advances render the mannitol Enzyme II the most amenable for study among the Enzymes II. Moreover, it is among the best characterized of permease proteins. The results reported here emphasize the multifunctional nature of the protein both in catalysis and regulation (Table 1). Further studies employing a combined genetic, biochemical, biophysical, and physiological approach should yield startling new insights into such related fields as membrane protein structure, permease function, chemoreception, transcriptional regulation, and the evolution of protein multifunctionality. The mannitol operon is likely to be at the forefront of membrane molecular biological research for many years to come.

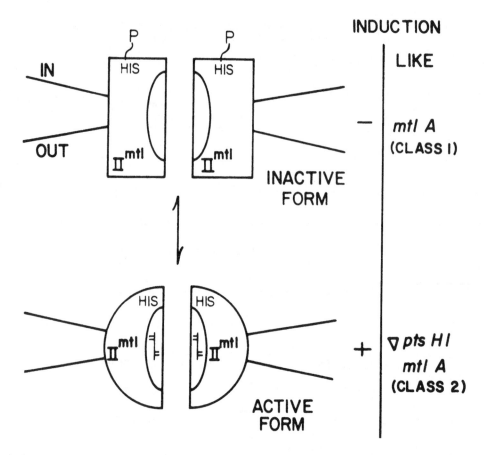

FIGURE 11.   Schematic depiction of two conformations of the Enzyme II^{Mtl} which may differentially affect transcription of the *mtl* operon. See text for details.

ACKNOWLEDGMENTS

We thank Cathy Lee and Gary Jacobson for valuable discussions and for permission to include in this review and discuss some of their unpublished results. Personal communication of unpublished results by Drs. P. V. Phibbs and B. N. Waygood are also gratefully acknowledged. Work in the authors' laboratory was supported by PHS grant 2 RO1 AI 14170-01 from the National Institute of Allergy and Infectious Diseases.

REFERENCES

1. **Stadtman, E. R.,** Allosteric regulation of enzyme activity, *Adv. Enzymol.*, 28, 42, 1966.
2. **Hatfield, D., Hofnung, M., and Schwartz, M.,** Nonsense mutations in the maltose A region of the genetic map of *Escherichia coli, J. Bacteriol.*, 100, 1311, 1969.
3. **Simoni, R. D. and Roseman, S.,** Sugar transport. VII. Lactose transport in *Staphylococcus aureus, J. Biol. Chem.*, 248, 966, 1973.
4. **Saier, M. H., Jr.,** The role of the cell surface in regulating the internal environment, in *The Bacteria*, Vol. 6, Sokatch, J. R. and Ornstein, L. N., Eds., Academic Press, New York, 1979, 167.

5. **Dills, S. S., Apperson, A., Schmidt, M. R., and Saier, M. H., Jr.,** Carbohydrate transport in bacteria, *Microbiol. Rev.,* 44, 385, 1980.

6. **Jacobson, G. R., Lee, C. A., and Saier, M. H., Jr.,** Purification of the mannitol-specific enzyme II of the *Escherichia coli* phosphoenolpyruvate: sugar phosphotransferase system, *J. Biol. Chem.,* 254, 249, 1979.

7. **Lee, C. A., Jacobson, G. R., and Saier, M. H., Jr.,** Plasmid-directed synthesis of the enzymes required for D-mannitol transport and utilization in *Escherichia coli, Proc. Natl. Acad. Sci.,* 78, 7336, 1981.

8. **Saier, M. H., Jr., Simoni, R. D., and Roseman, S.,** Sugar transport. Properties of mutant bacteria defective in proteins of the phosphoenolpyruvate: sugar phosphotransferase system, *J. Biol. Chem.,* 251, 6584, 1976.

9. **Saier, M. H., Jr., Simoni, R. D., and Roseman, S.,** The physiological behavior of Enzyme I and heat stable protein mutants of a bacterial phosphotransferase system, *J. Biol. Chem.,* 245, 5870, 1970.

10. **Cordaro, J. C., Anderson, R. P., Grogan, E. W., Jr., Wenzel, D.J., Engler, M., and Roseman, S.,** Promoter-like mutation affecting HPr and Enzyme I of the phosphoenolpyruvate:sugar phosphotransferase system in *Salmonella typhimurium, J. Bacteriol.,* 120, 245, 1974.

11. **Berkowitz, D.,** D-mannitol utilization in *Salmonella typhimurium, J. Bacteriol.,* 105, 232, 1971.

12. **Lengeler, J. and Steinberger, H.,** Analysis of the regulatory mechanisms controlling the synthesis of the hexitol transport systems in *Escherichia coli* K12, *Mol. Gen. Genet.,* 164, 163, 1978.

13. **Lengeler, J. and Steinberger, H.,** Analysis of regulatory mechanisms controlling the activity of the hexitol transport systems in *Escherichia coli* K12, *Mol. Gen. Genet.,* 167, 75, 1978.

14. **Adler, J. and Epstein, W.,** Phosphotransferase system enzymes as chemoreceptors for certain sugars in *E. coli* chemotaxis, *Proc. Natl. Acad. Sci. U.S.A.,* 71, 2895, 1974.

15. **Adler, J., Hazelbauer, G. L., and Dahl, M. M.,** Chemotaxis toward sugars in *Escherichia coli, J. Bacteriol.,* 115, 824, 1973.

16. **Melton, T., Hartman, P. E., Stratis, J.P., Lee, T. L., and Davis, A. T.,** Chemotaxis of *Salmonella typhimurium* to amino acids and some sugars, *J. Bacteriol.,* 133, 708, 1978.

17. **Saier, M. H., Jr. and Newman, M. J.,** Direct transfer of the phosphoryl moiety of mannitol 1-phosphate to [^{14}C]mannitol catalyzed by the Enzyme II complexes of the phosphoenolpyruvate:mannitol phosphotransferase systems in *Spirochaeta aurantia* and *Salmonella typhimurium, J. Biol. Chem.,* 251, 3834, 1976.

18. **Leonard, J. E., Lee, C. A., Apperson, A., Dills, S. S., and Saier, M. H., Jr.,** The role of membranes in the transport of small molecules, in *Membrane Structures in Bacterial Cells,* Vol. 1, Ghosh, B. K., Ed., CRC Press, Boca Raton, Florida, 1981, 1.

19. **Saier, M. H., Jr.,** Catalytic activities associated with the Enzymes II of the bacterial phosphotransferase system, *J. Supramol. Struct.,* 14, 281, 1981.

20. **Rephaeli, A. W. and Saier, M. H., Jr.,** Kinetic analyses of the sugar phosphate:sugar transphosphorylation reaction catalyzed by the glucose Enzyme II complex of the bacterial phosphotransferase system, *J. Biol. Chem.,* 253, 7595, 1978.

21. **Rephaeli, A. W. and Saier, M. H., Jr.,** Substrate specificity and kinetic characterization of sugar uptake and phosphorylation, catalyzed by the mannose Enzyme II of the phosphotransferase system in *Salmonella typhimurium, J. Biol. Chem.,* 255, 8585, 1980.

22. **Saier, M. H., Jr. and Schmidt, M. R.,** Vectorial and nonvectorial transphosphorylation catalyzed by Enzymes II of the bacterial phosphotransferase system, *J. Bacteriol.,* 145, 391, 1981.

23. **Haguenauer-Tsapis, R. and Kepes, A.,** Different sidedness of functionally homologous essential thiols in two membrane-bound phosphotransferase enzymes of *Escherichia coli* detected by permeant and non-permeant thiol reagents, *J. Biol. Chem.,* 255, 5075, 1980.

24. **Saier, M. H., Jr., Feucht, B. U., and Mora, W. K.,** Sugar phosphate:sugar transphosphorylation and exchange group translocation catalyzed by the Enzyme II complexes of the bacterial phosphoenolpyruvate:sugar phosphotransferase system, *J. Biol. Chem.,* 252, 8899, 1977.

25. **Singer, S. J.,** Thermodynamics, the structure of integral membrane proteins, and transport, *J. Supramol. Struct.,* 6, 313, 1977.

26. **Saier, M. H., Jr.,** Bacterial phosphoenolpyruvate:sugar phosphotransferase systems: structural, functional, and evolutionary inter-relationships, *Bacteriol. Rev.,* 41, 856, 1977.

27. **Saier, M. H., Jr., Feucht, B. U., and Roseman, S.,** Phosphoenolpyruvate-dependent fructose phosphorylation in photosynthetic bacteria, *J. Biol. Chem.,* 246, 7819, 1971.

28. **Saier, M. H., Jr., Newman, M. J., and Rephaeli, A. W.,** Properties of a phosphoenolpyruvate:mannitol phosphotransferase system in *Spirochaeta aurantia, J. Biol. Chem.,* 252, 8890, 1977.

29. **White, R. J. and Kent, P. W.,** An examination of the inhibitory effects of *N*-Iodoacetylglucosamine on *Escherichia coli* and isolation of resistant mutants, *Biochem. J.,* 118, 81, 1970.

30. **White, R. J.,** The role of the phosphoenolpyruvate phosphotransferase system in the transport of *N*-acetyl-D-glucosamine by *Escherichia coli, Biochem. J.,* 118, 89, 1970.

31. **Rose, S. P. and Fox, C. F.,** The β-glucoside system of *Escherichia coli* III. Properties of a P:HPr:β-glucoside phosphotransferase extracted from membranes with detergent, *J. Supramol. Struct.,* 1, 565, 1973.

32. **Rephaeli, A. W. and Saier, M. H., Jr.,** Regulation of genes coding for enzyme constituents of the bacterial phosphotransferase system, *J. Bacteriol.,* 141, 658, 1980.

33. **Riley, M. and Anilionis, A.,** Evolution of the bacterial genome, *Annu. Rev. Microbiol.,* 32, 519, 1978.

34. **Jones-Mortimer, M. C. and Kornberg, H. L.,** Uptake of fructose by the sorbitol phosphotransferase of *Escherichia coli* K12, *J. Gen. Microbiol.,* 96, 383, 1976.

35. **Conrad, R. and Schlegel, H. G.,** Different pathways for fructose and glucose utilization in *Rhodopseudomonas capsulata* and demonstration of 1-phosphofructokinase in phototropic bacteria, *Biochim. Biophys. Acta,* 358, 221, 1974.

36. **Sawyer, M. H., Baumann, P., and Baumann, L.,** Pathways of D-fructose and D-glucose catabolism in marine species of *Alcaligenes, Pseudomonas marina,* and *Alteromonas communis, Arch. Microbiol.,* 112, 169, 1977.

37. **Phibbs, P. V., Jr., McCowen, S. M., Feary, T. W., and Blevins, W. T.,** Mannitol and fructose catabolic pathways of *Pseudomonas aeruginosa* carbohydrate-negative mutants and pleiotropic effects of certain enzyme deficiencies, *J. Bacteriol.,* 133, 717, 1978.

38. **Sawyer, M. H., Baumann, P., Baumann, L., Berman, S.M., Canovas, J. L., and Berman, R. H.,** Pathways of D-fructose catabolism in species of *Pseudomonas, Arch. Microbiol.,* 112, 49, 1977.

39. **Reeves, R. E., Warren, L. G., and Hsu, D. S.,** 1-Phosphofructokinase from an anaerobe, *J. Biol. Chem.,* 241, 1257, 1966.

40. **Englesberg, E., Watson, J. A., and Hoffee, P. A.,** The glucose effect and the relationship between glucose permease, acid phosphatase, and glucose resistance, *Cold Spring Harbor Symp. Quant. Biol.,* 26, 261, 1961.

41. **Englesber G., E.,** Glucose inhibition and the diauxie phenomenon, *Proc. Natl. Acad. Sci.,* 45, 1494, 1959.

42. **Leonard, J. E. and Saier, M. H., Jr.,** Genetic dissection of catalytic activities of the *Salmonella typhimurium* mannitol Enzyme II, *J. Bacteriol.,* 145, 1106, 1981.

43. **Yashphe, J. and Kaplan, N. O.,** Revertants of *Escherichia coli* mutants defective in the cyclic AMP system, *Arch. Biochem. Biophys.,* 167, 388, 1975.

44. **Csonka, L. N. and Clark, A. J.,** Deletions generated by the transposon Tn10 in the *srl recA* region of the *Escherichia coli* K-12 chromosome, *Genetics,* 93, 321, 1979.

45. **Kundig, W. and Roseman, S.,** Sugar transport. I. Isolation of a phosphotransferase system from *Escherichia coli, J. Biol. Chem.,* 246, 1393, 1971.

46. **Anderson, B., Weigel, N., Kundig, W., and Roseman, S.,** Sugar transport. III. Purification and properties of a phosphocarrier protein (HPr) of the phosphoenolpyruvate-dependent phosphotransferase system of Escherichia coli, *J. Biol. Chem.,* 246, 7023, 1971.

47. **Jacobson, G. R.,** unpublished results.

48. **Jacobson, G. R., Lee, C. A., Leonard, J. E., and Saier, M. H., Jr.,** unpublished results.

49. **Leonard, J. E.,** unpublished results.

50. **Jacobson, G. R. and Saier, M. H., Jr.,** unpublished results.

51. **Phibbs, P. V.,** personal communication.

52. **Waygood, B.N.,** personal communication.

53. **Lee, C. A. and Saier, M. H., Jr.,** unpublished results.

54. **Lee, C. A. and Corbin, D. R.,** unpublished results.

Chapter 3

ESCHERICHIA COLI RIBOSOMAL PROTEINS INVOLVED IN AUTOGENOUS REGULATION OF TRANSLATION

John Yates and Masayasu Nomura

TABLE OF CONTENTS

I. INTRODUCTION

Ribosomes are the supramolecular structures that provide the site for, and participate in, the catalysis of protein synthesis.[1] The *Escherichia coli* ribosome is composed of two-thirds RNA (rRNA) and one-third protein (r-protein) by mass. Most of the r-proteins are small (average molecular weight about 15,000), basic and are present in a single copy per ribosome (L7/L12 being an exception, present in four copies).* Each ribosome consists of a small subunit containing 21 unique r-proteins bound to a 16S rRNA molecule, and a large subunit containing 31 unique r-proteins bound to single 23S and 5S rRNA molecules. Thus, the complexity of ribosomes can be appreciated not only in terms of their structure and function in relation to protein synthesis but also in terms of the genetic organization and physiological regulation of genes coding for ribosomal components.

In exponentially growing *E. coli* cells the synthetic rate for most, if not all, r-proteins is identical to the rate of accumulation of mature ribosomes.[2-4] Therefore "free" r-proteins do not accumulate nor is there significant degradation of r-proteins. Moreover, the synthesis of rRNA and r-proteins is coordinately regulated in response to environmental changes. How is this remarkable regulation accomplished? We have recently proposed that r-protein synthesis and RNA synthesis are coupled, and that r-proteins not sequestered by rRNA into ribosomal particles can prevent their own synthesis by inhibition of the further translation of their own mRNA.[5] Thus some r-proteins have a physiological role in regulating gene expression in addition to their roles in the assembly, structure, and function of the ribosome. In this article we discuss experiments that confirm and extend the model for autogenous translational regulation of r-protein synthesis.

II. ORGANIZATION AND EXPRESSION OF r-PROTEIN GENES IN *E. coli*

Ribosomal protein genes are organized into at least 16 distinct transcriptional units scattered about the *E. coli* chromosome.[6,7] Twenty-seven r-protein genes are clustered within four operons located in the 72 min region of the chromosome. These operons, called the *str*, *spc*, *S10*, and α operons, encode from 2 to 11 unique r-proteins each. The "*rif*" cluster at 77 min contains another four r-protein genes in the β and L11 operons. In some cases r-protein operons also contain other genes related to the transcription and translation process. The structures of the above operons are shown in Figure 1.[7] The elucidation of the structures of the r-protein operons was accomplished by the isolation and subsequent biochemical and genetic analysis of transducing phages that carry r-protein genes. The 27 r-protein genes in the 72 min region were originally isolated as transducing phage λ*fus 3*[8] and subsets of these genes were isolated as λ*spc1* and λ *spc2*.[9] The "*rif* " cluster of four r-protein genes were identified on λ*rif* ^d18[10,11] which was originally isolated as a phage carrying genes for RNA polymerase subunits β and βc'.[12]

The availability of transducing phages carrying r-protein genes has greatly facilitated the study of r-protein gene expression. It was found that lysogens of λ*spc1*, merodiploid for r-protein genes of the α and *spc* operons, synthesized the r-proteins from these operons at the same rate as the other r-proteins whose genes were in single copies in the cell. However, when mRNA synthesis rates were measured, by using DNA from the transducing phages as hybridization probes, increased transcription rates in proportion to the increase in gene dosage of the r-protein genes were observed. From these studies, a model was proposed that r-protein synthesis is feedback regulated at a posttranscriptional level.[5]

---

* L7 is an N-acetylated derivative of protein L12. "L7/L12" refers to the mixture of the two forms of the protein.

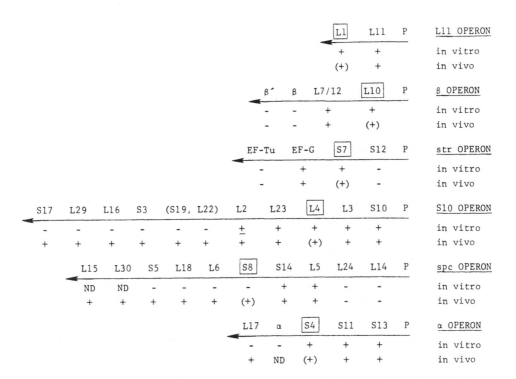

FIGURE 1. Autogenous regulation of r-protein genes of *E. coli* located in the *str-spc* and *rif* chromosomal regions. Genes are represented by the protein product. For each operon, the order of transcription from the promoter (P) is indicated by an arrow. Regulatory r-proteins are indicated by the boxes. Effects of the boxed protein on the in vitro or in vivo synthesis of proteins from the same operon are shown. Results obtained in vivo are those from experiments using hybrid plasmids to achieve overproduction of the regulatory r-protein. (+) specific inhibition of synthesis; (−) no significant effect on synthesis; (±) weak specific inhibition observed in vitro; (+) inhibition presumed to occur in vivo; (ND) not determined.

III. MECHANISMS OF AUTOGENOUS REGULATION OF r-PROTEIN SYNTHESIS

Several r-proteins were subsequently shown to inhibit autogenously r-protein synthesis both in vitro and in vivo. Synthesis of r-proteins was carried out in vitro using DNA of λ*spc1*, λ*fus 3* and λ*rif* [d]18 transducing phages as templates. Individual purified r-proteins were tested in vitro for effects on r-protein synthesis when added directly to the protein synthesizing system. We found that six r-proteins, S4, S7, S8, L1, L4, and L10, cause specific inhibition of their own synthesis and the inhibition of the synthesis of other proteins contained within their own operons (see Figure 1), and that this inhibition is exerted at the level of mRNA translation.[13-16] Other researchers have independently discovered the regulatory effects of L10 in vitro.[17,18] In vitro experiments of Wirth and Böck[19,20] indicate that S20 similarly feedback regulates its own synthesis.

The regulatory properties of many r-proteins have also been determined in vivo, by using recombinant plasmids in which r-protein genes were fused to the regulatory elements of the lactose or arabinose operon. Excess synthesis of specific r-proteins could then be induced in the cells by the addition of an inducer of the lactose or arabinose operon to the culture of cells. Using this method, we confirmed the in vitro identification of S4, S7, S8, L1, and L10 as regulatory r-proteins in their respective operons,[15,16,21,22] while Lindahl and co-workers[23,24] independently identified L4 as the regulatory r-protein of the S10 operon. The results of these investigations are summarized in Figure 1. S7, S8, and L10 inhibit the in vivo synthesis of some, but not all of the proteins from their operons, consistent with the in vitro observation that these r-proteins regulate mRNA translation, and not transcription. As shown in Figure 1, inhibition of r-protein synthesis in vivo by S4, S8, and L4 extends distally to the ends of these operons, while the in vitro synthesis of the distal proteins was not affected. One possible explanation for this discrepancy is that large polycistronic mRNAs become fragmented in vitro (but not in vivo), and the mRNA molecules that have lost the promoter proximal control regions give rise to the weak synthesis, insensitive to repression, that we observe (see discussion of repression of translation of polycistronic mRNA below.)

We refer to a group of proteins whose genes are clustered in an operon and translationally regulated by one member of the group as a regulatory unit. In some cases (e.g., the L11 and S10 operons), one regulatory unit encompasses the entire operon, while other operons (the *spc*, *str*, and β operons) are divided into units of regulation. No r-protein that is under the translational control of another r-protein has been found to have an autoregulatory capacity; that is, translational regulatory units have not been found to overlap. The existence of these units of regulation raises two questions about the mechanisms involved in expression of r-protein genes. First, how does a repressor r-protein block translation of several cistrons of a polycistronic mRNA? Secondly, what mechanisms ensure that the r-proteins within regulatory units are synthesized in the correct ratio?

The mechanism of r-protein repressor action has been most extensively studied with r-protein L1 of the L11 operon. The L11 operon consists of genes for two r-proteins, L11 and L1, with the synthesis of both proteins being feedback regulated by L1. In studying translational repression using a DNA-dependent in vitro system, DNA templates were used that bisect the L11 operon near the 5′ end in order to produce mRNA from the corresponding portions of the operon. It was found that the first 160 bases from the 5′ end of the mRNA contain a functional target site for L1 repressor action, and that the remainder of the mRNA of the operon lacked an independent site for translational repression.[25] Thus, it was concluded that the synthesis of both proteins L11 and L1 from the bicistronic mRNA is repressed by L1 action at the translation initiation site for L11 synthesis, and that, in the absence of translation of the L11 mRNA, the distal L1 mRNA cannot be translated. This conclusion, considered with the fact that L11 and L1 are synthesized at equimolar rates in vivo, has led us to propose that L11 and L1 mRNA are sequentially translated by the same ribosomes.[25] Thus, only the translation initiation site for L11 synthesis can serve as the entry site for free ribosomes to bind to the bicistronic mRNA and begin translation. Then following termination of the L11 polypeptide chain, the same ribosomes (or ribosomal components, e.g., 30S subunit) would reinitiate and translate the L1 coding sequence of the mRNA. This process, which we call "sequential translation" (of a cluster of cistrons within a polycistronic mRNA) allows for translational regulation of the synthesis of a group of proteins as a unit using a single regulatory site on the mRNA, while additionally ensuring that all proteins within the regulatory unit are synthesized in equimolar amounts.

A general feature of feedback regulation of r-protein synthesis appears to be the location of the repressor target sites at the 5′ end of the regulatory unit. For all known repressor r-proteins except S7 and S8, the target sites are located near the 5′ ends of the respective mRNA transcripts. With S7 and S8, whose regulatory units do not include the most promoter-proximal genes of the operons, the target sites appear to involve the regions of mRNA around the translational initiation sites of the first cistrons of their regulatory units.[26,27] As in the case of the L11 operon, translation of distal cistrons within a regulatory unit appears to depend on translation of the first cistron of the group. Since all of the proteins of these regulatory units (except L7/L12, see below) are synthesized in the equimolar ratios of one copy per ribosome, the sequential translational model could apply to these regulatory units as well as to the L11 operon.

An alternative model for the expression of ribosomal proteins within translational regulatory units is that translation of each cistron can be initiated by free ribosomes: but, the initiation at second and more distal cistrons depends on the translation a certain distance into the preceeding cistron, which is required to disrupt secondary or tertiary mRNA structures that otherwise prevent access of ribosomes to the initiation sites. Independent initiation would only occur at the start site of the first cistron of the regulatory unit. The ratio of proteins synthesized in the regulatory unit would depend on the relative strengths of initiation signals at the different translation start sites on the polycistronic mRNA. Such a model could be required to account for regulation of L7/L12 synthesis by L10. L10 translationally represses the synthesis of both L10 and L7/L12, the products of the first and second genes, respectively, of the β operon (see Figure 1). Yet while ribosomes contain a single copy of L10 (like almost all other ribosomal proteins), they contain four copies of L7/L12.[28,29] In vitro experiments demonstrate that the L10 target site is at the beginning of the L10 gene and that there is no independent site for repressor action near the L7/L12 gene.[16] The results imply that translation of L7/L12 mRNA, though at least four times as efficient as translation of L10 mRNA, is nevertheless dependent upon translation of the preceeding L10 mRNA.

Oppenheim and Yanofsky[30] have found from their studies on the *trp* operon that *trpD* translation is dependent upon translation of the upstream *trpE* mRNA and termed this phenomenon "translational coupling." With this terminology, we can say that r-protein synthesis within translational regulatory units is translationally coupled. Within regulatory units in which the proteins are synthesized in equimolar amounts, we think it is likely that translation of cistrons is sequential, as well. If L7/L12 does not exert independent feedback inhibition upon its own synthesis (there is no evidence to indicate that it does), then the ratio of L10 to L7/L12 synthesized from the L10-L7/L12 mRNA would reflect the relative strengths of the translation initiation signals for the two genes. We might expect that if the translation initiation signals are not exactly tuned, there may be an excess of L7/L12 synthesis. There have been reports[31,32] that excess L7/L12 synthesis occurs in vivo, and that unlike other r-proteins, significant amount of L7/L12 can be detected free of ribosomes.

One conceivable mechanism for repressor r-proteins to inhibit synthesis from large regulatory units is the repression of translation initiation at a cistron, causing termination of transcription within that cistron, and thereby, preventing the expression of all the distal cistrons of the operon. In one case, that of feedback repression by L4 in the S10 operon, oversynthesis of L4 in vivo does cause a marked decrease in the rate of mRNA synthesis from the operon.[24] Such a mechanism of transcription termination caused by repression of translation could therefore apply to feedback regulation of S10 operon expression. However, this postulated mechanism does not appear to be the general one. First, it was observed that in strains carrying extra gene copies in the *spc* and α operons, the rate of transcription increases (the rate of translation does not increase) in proportion to the increase in gene copy numbers.[5,33] Similar observations were made for expression of the β operon[34] and of the S1 gene.[35] Second, in the *str* (or β) operon, overproduction of the repressor protein S7 (or L10) from a fusion operon did not cause a decrease in the synthesis of Tu (or β and β') from the distal part of the operon. Therefore, the repressor does not appear to cause transcription termination in such a case. Finally, it should also be pointed out that even for the S10 operon, specific translational repression of four to five promoter proximal genes by the repressor L4 was observed in the absence of transcription in vitro. Such in vitro effects cannot be explained by the postulated transcriptional mechanism. Therefore, we think that sequential translation (or translational coupling) occurs in the S10 operon as in other operons.

IV. REPRESSOR ACTION AT mRNA TARGET SITES

All repressor r-proteins identified thus far bind independently to specific regions of rRNA,

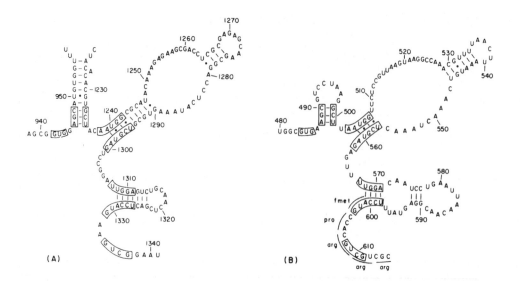

FIGURE 2.   Model of the secondary structure of the S7 binding sites on 16S rRNA (A) and on mRNA (B). Boxed sequences indicate homology. The structure of part of 16S rRNA shown in (A) is taken from Reference 64. [S7 has been crosslinked by ultraviolet irradiation to the U at position 1240.[65,66]] In (B) the S12 coding region ends at 501, and the S7 coding region begins at 604. The mRNA sequence is taken from Reference 67.

and are among the "initial binding proteins" in the in vitro assembly of ribosomes. Feedback regulation involving these r-proteins can then be regarded as competition between mRNA and rRNA for binding of the repressor r-proteins. We have in fact observed that the presence of 23S rRNA during in vitro protein synthesis can abolish the repressor activity of L1.[25] Similarly, the evidence that S20 is an autoregulatory protein is that the presence of 16S rRNA, to which S20 binds, specifically stimulates in vitro synthesis of S20. L10 has been shown to bind to L10 mRNA near the 5' end,[70] and 23S rRNA competes for this binding. A simple way for such a feedback regulatory mechanism to arise through evolution would be for the mRNA to develop, near its translational initiation region, similarities to the binding site on rRNA for the r-protein that the mRNA encodes. For those repressor r-proteins whose rRNA binding sites are known, we have found that structural homologies between the rRNA binding sites and the putative mRNA target sites do in fact exist.[26,27]

Figures 2 and 3 illustrate a comparison of the 16S rRNA binding sites for S7 and S8 with the mRNA around the translational start sites for the first proteins, S7 and L5, endoded in their respective regulatory units. The 16S rRNA binding sites for S7 and S8 have been well characterized, and therefore, it is possible to make meaningful comparison of mRNA target sites with the rRNA binding sites. It can be seen that, in each case, several runs of nucleotides three to eight nucleotides long occur in both mRNA and rRNA in the same order and with similar spacing in the sequences. In addition, the mRNAs can be represented, as in Figures 2 and 3, with secondary structures that are homologous to the secondary structures that are believed to exist in the 16S rRNA. For the mRNA target sites of both S7 and S8, the AUG initiation codons are within regions of both primary and secondary structural homology to the corresponding 16S rRNA binding sites. Presumably, binding of S7 and S8 to the mRNA target sites stabilizes these secondary structures and renders the AUG inaccessible to initiating ribosomes. We note that the homologous secondary structures for mRNA are expected to be unstable. Thus, in the absence of repressor r-protein, these secondary structures would not interfere with translation initiation.

Target sites for S4 and L1 also share significant structural homology, with the corre-

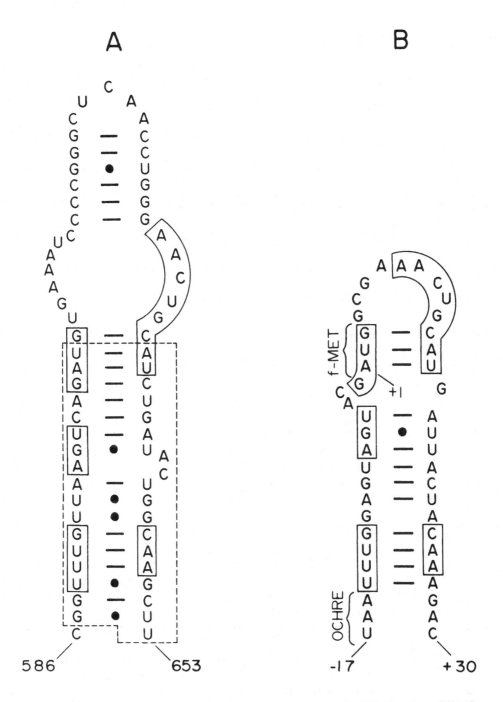

FIGURE 3. Model of the secondary structure of S8 binding sites on 16S rRNA (A) and on mRNA (B). Homologies which are considered to be significant are boxed. The structure shown in (A) is taken from Reference 64. The binding site for S8[68,69] is indicated by a broken line. In (B) the L24 coding region ends at −18, and the L5 coding region begins at +4. The mRNA sequence is taken from Reference 27.

sponding rRNA binding sites.[26,36,37] The same general features discussed above for the S7 and S8 target sites apply:

1.   Homology is observed in runs of nucleotide sequence and in secondary structure.

2.   Translational initiation sites are included within homologous secondary structures, which would be expected to be unstable in the absence of repressor r-protein.

The two remaining repressor r-proteins that we have studied, L4 and L10, have not been sufficiently characterized to facilitate comparisons with the mRNA and 23S rRNA target sites. However, it is likely that homology exists between rRNA and mRNA for the binding sites of these proteins as well, and preliminary inspection of the RNA sequences supports this notion. We expect that in a growing culture of *E. coli* the partitioning of repressor r-proteins between ribosome assembly and mRNA binding strongly favors the ribosome assembly reaction. Thus, feedback inhibition is only exerted by repressor r-proteins that are synthesized in excess over rRNA synthesis. All of the repressor r-proteins we have identified bind strongly and independently to rRNA. It is likely that the affinity of these repressor r-proteins for rRNA is greater than for mRNA. This difference in binding affinity suffices to ensure that ribosome assembly proceeds preferentially to mRNA binding. While comparative mRNA and rRNA binding experiments under the same conditions are needed, the limited information we have on r-protein-RNA interaction supports this notion.* The structural homologies between mRNA and rRNA, then, are probably a subset of those structural features of rRNA that comprise the r-protein binding sites. The instability of the base-paried stems of the S7 mRNA target site, for example, may result in the postulated lower affinity compared to that of 16S rRNA for binding S7.

It should be pointed out that the association of many r-proteins with rRNA is a highly cooperative process, and this cooperation should also ensure that repressor r-proteins take part in ribosome assembly preferential to mRNA binding. For example, L10, though able to bind to a specific fragment of 23S rRNA in the absence of any other r-proteins, is aided by L11, while L11 binding to the same RNA fragment is stimulated by L10.[39] Similarly, the binding of S7 to 16S rRNA is stimulated by some other r-proteins, e.g., S19 or S9.[40] Thus a ribosomal protein that has a rather low affinity for rRNA could still have sufficiently strong interaction with its mRNA for feedback inhibition of translation, and could rely on its cooperative interactions with other r-proteins to increase its affinity for rRNA or ribosome assembly intermediates over its affinity for mRNA.

V. SOME COMMENTS ON THE ROLES OF REGULATORY r-PROTEINS IN THE STRUCTURE AND FUNCTION OF RIBOSOMES

The striking homology observed to exist between rRNA binding sites and mRNA target sites of repressor r-proteins imply that the same regions of the protein molecules are involved in the interaction with both rRNA and mRNA. It is the property of site-specific interaction with RNA that allows these r-proteins to participate both in the function of ribosomes and in feedback regulation.

However, one can imagine that these r-proteins must have functions other than rRNA binding, and such functions may involve regions of the protein molecules different from those involved in the interaction with rRNA and mRNA. We shall consider this point using L10 and S4 as examples.

As mentioned above, L10 feedback regulates the synthesis of L7/L12 as well as its own

---

*   Association constants for binding of 16S RNA by S4 and S8 have been reported to be about 3.5×10^6 M^{-1} and 4×10^7 M^{-1}, respectively, under conditions of ribosome reconstitution,[34] while the concentrations required for half maximal inhibition of the synthesis of r-proteins in vitro indicate apparent association constants of approximately 1×10^6 M^{-1} for both S4 and S8 under conditions of lower ionic strength. We expect that the association constants for mRNA would be even lower under the conditions of higher ionic strength used for ribosome reconstitution.

synthesis from the bicistronic mRNA. One clearly established function of L10 in the ribosome is to hold L7/L12[41] which is directly involved in the binding of elongation factors EF-G and EF-Tu as well as initiation factor IF-2.[42] It is known that in solution[39,44] as well as in ribosomes,[29] L10 interacts directly with L7/L12. Four copies of L7/L12 exist on the 50S subunit of ribosomes, appearing to protrude from the 50S subunit as an elongated "stalk" in electron micrographs.[45] The four L7/L12 molecules bind via their amino terminal regions[46] to L10 which, in turn, binds to 50S ribosomes by interacting with 23S rRNA and, perhaps, L11 and other proteins. The functional regions of the L10 molecules appear to be the carboxy-terminal portion of the protein for binding L7/L12 and the amino terminus for binding 23S rRNA.[47] Because both free L10 and L10-L7/L12 complexes are equally active as translational repressors in vitro (our unpublished experiments), it is likely that the region of L10 involved in the interaction with L7/L12 (carboxy-terminal portion) is probably not essential for repression or interaction with 23S rRNA. Thus, the L10 molecule can be subdivided into two functional domains.

S4 is known to play a central role in organizing ribosome structure.[48] S4, like S7 or S8, is required for the binding of several other r-proteins during the reconstitution of 30S subunits.[40,49] It is likely that S4 interacts with one or several other r-proteins as well as with rRNA. S4, in fact, is buried in the 30S ribosomes by the presence of S5 and S12, at least to the extent that it is inaccessible to anti-S4 immunoglobulin.[50] Several experimental results suggest that: (1) the N-terminal portion of the molecule is required for binding several other r-proteins, but is not required for binding to 16S rRNA (and hence, presumably to mRNA target sites); (2) the C-terminal portion of the molecule is essential for binding to 16S rRNA and also to mRNA target sites. First, removal of N-terminal 46 amino acids from the 203 residue protein by mild trypsin digestion did not abolish 16S rRNA binding activity, but the use of this altered S4 in ribosome reconstitution resulted in the formation of particles deficient in several r-proteins (S1, S2, S10, S18 and S21).[51] Second, S4 molecules with up to 20% of the protein missing from the C-terminal end have been obtained through genetic mutations, mutations that suppress a phenotype of streptomycin-dependence.[52,53] Loss of carboxy-terminal regions of S4 in such mutants prevents ribosome assembly and cellular growth at high temperatures.[54] Such strains also oversynthesize proteins of the S4 regulatory unit, S11, S13, and S4, suggesting the involvement of the carboxy-terminal region of the S4 polypeptide in binding to its mRNA.[55,71] In merodiploid strains carrying both mutant and wild type S4 alleles, only the wild type S4 molecule is incorporated into ribosomes while the truncated S4 protein is degraded.[54] Thus, the carboxy-terminus of S4 probably contributes to the binding to 16S rRNA as well as to mRNA. Therefore, it appears that the S4 molecule is also subdivided into functionally different domains.

Although there is much information on the role of r-proteins with respect to the overall structural organization of the ribosomes, very little is known about the precise role of most of the r-proteins in protein synthesis. We believe (and there is some evidence) that at least some of the r-proteins are directly involved in the catalytic functions of ribosomes or in the interaction with other important soluble protein factors and substrate aminoacyl tRNAs (e.g., L7/L12, see above). On the other hand, it is also conceivable that some other r-proteins are mostly required for the assembly of the structure of ribosomes and not directly for function in protein synthesis. Some of the repressor r-proteins, such as L1 and S20, may belong to this class. This conclusion is based on mutant strains that have been found to lack each of these proteins. A phenotypic revertant of a kasugamycin dependent strain, already carrying at least two mutations, affecting L23 and methylation of 16S rRNA, was isolated that lacks detectable L1 protein.[56] Ribosomes which do not contain L1 are apparently functional,[57] and therefore, L1 does not appear to be essential in the context of certain other alterations in ribosome structure. As expected, the regulatory function of L1 was apparently absent in this mutant, resulting in the oversynthesis of L11.[58,59] The mutant also shows impaired growth rate. It is not known whether the slow growth rate results from an impaired (unknown) function of ribosomes resulting from the loss of L1; a decrease in the rate of assembly of ribosomes; the overproduction of L11 as a result of impaired regulation of its synthesis. Further studies may be able to indicate the relative importance of these functions of L1 for cellular growth. Similarly, mutants have been found that lack detectable protein S20.[60,61]

VI. CONCLUSIONS

Certain ribosomal proteins of *E. coli* function as translational repressors and regulate the translation of their own mRNA. Thus, these proteins have dual functional roles: the newly discovered regulatory role and the classical roles in the assembly and function of the ribosome. These two functional roles are not unrelated. The repressor function utilizes the protein's ability to perform a classical function, that is, to recognize specific structural features of rRNA. In this sense, the repressor r-proteins resemble the T4 gene 32 protein[62,63] (see also Chapter 4), and differs from some other multi-functional proteins which have several different functional domains with unrelated enzymatic activities. The feedback regulatory mechanism which evolved ensures the balanced and coordinated synthesis of many r-proteins, regulation which is probably vital for cellular growth. The present system may serve as a model system for regulation of synthesis of r-proteins in other organisms and of the coordination of synthesis of components of other supramolecular structures as well.

ACKNOWLEDGMENTS

This work was supported in part by the College of Agricultural and Life Sciences, University of Wisconsin, Madison, by Grant GM-20427 from the National Institutes of Health, and by Grant PCM79-10616 from the National Science Foundation. This is paper No. 2532 from the Laboratory of Genetics, University of Wisconsin, Madison.

REFERENCES

1. **Nomura, M., Tissieres, A., and Lengyel, P.,** *Ribosomes,* Cold Spring Harbor Laboratory, Cold Spring Harbor, New York, 1974.
2. **Dennis, P. P.,** *In vivo* stability, maturation and relative synthesis rates of inidividual ribosomal proteins in *Escherichia coli* B/r, *J. Mol. Biol.,* 88, 25, 1974.
3. **Kjeldgaard, N. O. and Gausing, K.,** Regulation of biosynthesis of ribosomes, in *Ribosomes,* Nomura, M., Tissieres, A., and Lengyel, P., Eds., Cold Spring Harbor Laboratory, Cold Spring Harbor, New York, 1974, 369.
4. **Nomura, M., Morgan, E. A., and Jaskunas, S. R.,** Genetics of bacterial ribosomes, *Annu. Rev. Genet.,* 11, 297, 1977.
5. **Fallon, A. M., Jinks, C. S., Strycharz, G. D., and Nomura, M.,** Regulation of ribosomal protein synthesis in *Escherichia coli* by selective mRNA inactivation, *Proc. Natl. Acad. Sci. U.S.A.,* 76, 3411, 1979.
6. **Isono, K.,** Genetics of ribosomal proteins and their modifying and processing enzymes in *Escherichia coli,* in *Ribosomes,* Chambliss, G., Craven, G. R., Davies, J., Davis, K., Kahan, L., and Nomura, M., Eds., University Park Press, Baltimore, 1980, 641.
7. **Nomura, M. and Post, L.,** Organization of ribosomal genes and regulation of their expression in *Escherichia coli,* in *Ribosomes,* Chambliss, G. H., Craven, G. R., Davies, J. E., Kahan, L. and Nomura, M., Eds., University Park Press, Baltimore, 1980, 671.
8. **Jaskunas, S. R., Fallon, A. M., and Nomura, M.,** Identification and organization of ribosomal protein genes of *Escherichia coli* carried by λfus2 transducing phage, *J. Biol. Chem.,* 252, 7323, 1977.

9. **Jaskunas, S. R., Lindahl, L., and Nomura, M.,** Specialized transducing phages for ribosomal protein 38genes of *Escherichia coli, Proc. Natl. Acad. Sci. U.S.A.,* 72, 6, 1975.

10. **Lindahl, L., Jaskunas, S.R., Dennis, P. P., and Nomura, M.,** Cluster of genes in *Escherichia coli* for ribosomal proteins, ribosomal RNA, and RNA polymerse subunits, *Proc. Natl. Acad. Sci. U.S.A.,* 72, 2743, 1975.

11. **Watson, R. J., Parker, J., Fiil, N. P., Flaks, J.G., and Friesen, J. D.,** New chromosomal location for structural genes of ribosomal proteins, *Proc. Natl. Acad. Sci. U.S.A.,* 72, 2765, 1975.

12. **Kirschbaum, J. B. and Konrad, E. G.,** Isolation of a specialized lambda transducing bacteriophage carrying the beta subunit gene for *Escherichia coli* ribonucleic acid polymerase, *J. Bacteriol.,* 116, 517, 1973.

13. **Yates, J. L., Arfsten, A. E., and Nomura, M.,** *In vitro* expression of *Escherichia coli* ribosomal protein genes: autogenous inhibition of translation, *Proc. Natl. Acad. Sci. U.S.A.,* 77, 1837, 1980.

14. **Yates, J. L. and Nomura, M.,** *E. coli* ribosomal protein L4 is a feedback regulatory protein, *Cell,* 21, 517, 1980.

15. **Dean, D., Yates, J. L., and Nomura, M.,** Identification of ribosomal protein S7 as a repressor of translation within the *str* operon of *Escherichia coli, Cell,* 24, 413, 1981.

16. **Yates, J. L., Dean, D., Strycharz, W. A., and Nomura, M.,** *E. coli* ribosomal protein L10 inhibits translation of L10 and L7/L12 mRNAs by acting at a single site, *Nature,* 294, 190, 1981.

17. **Brot, N., Caldwell, D., and Weissbach, H.,** Autogenous control of *Escherichia coli* ribosomal protein L10 synthesis *in vitro, Proc. Natl. Acad. Sci. U.S.A.,* 77, 2592, 1980.

18. **Fukuda, R.,** Autogenous regulation of the synthesis of ribosomal proteins, L10 and L7/L12, *in Escherichia coli, Mol. Gen. Genet.,* 178, 483, 1980.

19. **Wirth, R. and Böck, A.,** Regulation of synthesis of ribosomal protein S20 *in vitro, Mol. Gen. Genet.,* 178, 479, 1980.

20. **Wirth, R., Kohler, V., and Böck, A.,** Factors modulating transcription and translation *in vitro* of ribosomal protein S20 and isoleucyl-tRNA synthetase from *Escherichia coli, Eur. J. Biochem.,* 114, 429, 1981.

21. **Dean, D. and Nomura, M.,** Feedback regulation of ribosomal protein gene expression in *Escherichia coli, Proc. Natl. Acad. Sci. U.S.A.,* 77, 3590, 1980.

22. **Dean, D., Yates, J. L., and Nomura, M.,** *Escherichia coli* ribosomal protein S8 feedback regulates part of the *spc* operon, *Nature,* 289, 89, 1981.

23. **Lindahl, L. and Zengel, J.,** Operon-specific regulation of ribosomal protein synthesis in *Escherichia coli, Proc. Natl. Acad. Sci. U.S.A.,* 76, 6542, 1979.

24. **Zengel, J. M., Meuckl, D., and Lindahl, L.,** Protein L4 of the *E. coli* ribosome regulates an eleven gene r protein operon, *Cell,* 21, 523, 1980.

25. **Yates, J. L. and Nomura, M.,** Feedback regulation of ribosomal protein synthesis in *E. coli:* localization of the mRNA target site for repressor action of ribosomal protein L1, *Cell,* 24, 243, 1981.

26. **Nomura, M., Yates, J. L., Dean, D., and Post, L. E.,** Feedback regulation of ribosomal protein gene expression in *Escherichia coli:* structural homology of ribosomal RNA and ribosomal protein mRNA, *Proc. Natl. Acad. Sci. U.S.A.,* 77, 7084, 1980.

27. **Olins, P. O. and Nomura, M.,** Translational regulation by ribosomal protein S8 in *Escherichia coli:* structural homology between rRNA binding site and feedback target on mRNA, *Nucleic Acids Res.,* 9, 1757, 1981.

28. **Hardy, S. J. J.,** The stoichiometry of the ribosomal proteins of *Escherichia coli, Mol. Gen. Genet.,* 140, 253, 1975.

29. **Marquis, D. and Fahnestock, S. R.,** A complex of acidic ribosomal proteins: evidence of a four-to-one complex of proteins in the Bacillus stearothermophilus ribosome, *J. Mol. Biol.,* 119, 557, 1978.

30. **Oppenheim, D. S. and Yanofsky, C.,** Translational coupling during expression of the tryotphan operon in *Escherichia coli, Genetics,* 95, 785, 1980.

31. **Morrissey, J. J., Weissbach, H., and Brot, N.,** The identification and characterization of proteins similar to L7, L12 in ribosome-free extracts of *Escherichia coli, Biochem. Biophys. Res. Commun.,* 65, 293, 1975.

32. **Morrissey, J. J., Cupp, L. E., Weissbach, H., and Brot, N.,** Synthesis of ribosomal proteins L7/L12 in related and stringent strains of *Escherichia coli, J. Biol. Chem.,* 251, 5516, 1976.

33. **Olsson, M. O. and Gausing, K.,** Post-transcriptional control of coordinated ribosomal protein synthesis in *Escherichia coli, Nature,* 283, 599, 1980.

34. **Dennis, P. P. and Fiil, N. P.,** Transcriptional and post-transcriptional control of RNA polymerase and ribosomal protein genes cloned on composite ColEl plasmids in the bacterium *Escherichia coli, J. Biol. Chem.,* 254, 7540, 1979.

35. **Christiansen, L. and Pederson, J.,** Cloning restriction endonuclease mapping and post-transcriptional regulation of rpsA, the structural gene for ribosomal protein S1, *Mol. Gen. Genet.,* 181, 548, 1981.

36. **Gourse, R. L., Thurlow, D. L., Gerbi, S. A., and Zimmerman, R. A.,** Specific binding of a prokaryotic ribosomal protein to a eukaryotic ribosomal RNA: implications for evolution and autoregulation, *Proc. Natl. Acad. Sci. U.S.A.,* 78, 2722, 1981.

37. **Branlant, C., Krol, A., Machatt, A., and Ebel, J. P.,** The secondary structure of the protein L1 binding region of ribosomal 23S RNA. Homologies with putative secondary structures of the L11 mRNA and of a region of mitochondrial 16S rRNA, *Nucleic Acids Res.,* 9, 293, 1981.

38. **Spicer, E., Schwarzbauer, J., and Craven, G. R.,** Isolation of ribosomal protein-RNA complexes by nitrocellulose membrane filtration: equilibrium binding studies, *Nucleic Acids Res.,* 4, 491, 1977.

39. **Dijk, J., Garrett, R.A., and Müller, R.,** Studies on the binding of the ribosomal complex L7/L12-L10 and protein L11 to the 5'-one third of 23S RNA: a functional centre of the 50S subunit, *Nucleic Acids Res.,* 6, 2717, 1979.

40. **Mizushima, S. and Nomura, M.,** Assembly mapping of 30S ribosomal proteins from *Escherichia coli,* *Nature,* 226, 1214, 1970.

41. **Highland, J. H. and Howard, G. A.,** Assembly of ribosomal proteins L7, L10, L11 and L12 on the 50S subunit of *Escherichia coli, J. Biol. Chem.,* 250, 831, 1975.

42. **Möller, W.,** The ribosomal components involved in EF-G- and EF-Tu-dependent GTP hydrolysis, in *Ribosomes,* Nomura, M., Tissieres, A., and Lengyel, P., Eds., Cold Spring Harbor Laboratory, New York, 1974, 711.

43. **Chu, F., Caldwell, P., Samuels, M., Weissbach, H., and Brot, N.,** NDA-dependent *in vitro* synthesis of *Escherichia coli* ribosomal protein L10 and the formation of an L10/L12 complex, *Biochem. Biophys. Res. Commun.,* 76, 593, 1977.

44. **Österberg, R., Sjöberg, B., Petterson, I., Liljas, A., and Kurland, C. G.,** Small-angle X-ray scattering study of the protein complex of L7/L12 and L10 from *Escherichia coli* ribosomes, *FEBS Lett.,* 73, 22, 1977.

45. **Strycharz, W. A., Nomura, M., and Lake, J. F.,** Ribosomal proteins L7/L12 localized at a single region of the large subunit by immune electron microscopy, *J. Mol. Biol.,* 126, 123, 1978.

46. **van Agthoven, A. J., Maassen, J. A., Schrier, P. I., and Möller, W.,** Inhibition of EF-G dependent GTPase by an aminoterminal fragment of L7/L12, *Biochem. Biophys. Res. Commun.,* 64, 1184, 1975.

47. **Gudkov, A. J., Tumanova, L. G., Gongadze, G. M., and Bushuev, V. N.,** Role of different regions of ribosomal proteins L7 and L10 in their complex formation and in the interaction with the ribosomal 50S subunit, *FEBS Lett.,* 109, 34, 1980.

48. **Zimmerman, R. A.,** Interaction among protein and RNA components of the ribosomes, in *Ribosomes,* Chambliss, G. H., Craven, G.R., Davies, J.E., Khan, L., and Nomura, M., Eds., University Park Press, Baltimore, 1980, 135.

49. **Nomura, M. and Held, W.A.,** Reconstitution of ribosomes: studies of ribosome structure, function, and assembly, in *Ribosomes,* Nomura, M., Tissieres, A., and Lengyel, P., Eds., Cold Spring Harbor Laboratory, Cold Spring Harbor, New York, 1974, 193.

50. **Winkleman, D. and Kahan, L.,** The reaction of antibodies with ribosomal subunits and assembly intermediates, in *Ribosomes,* Chambliss, G. H., Craven, G. R., Davies, J. E., Kahan, L., and Nomura, M., Eds., University Park Press, Baltimore, 1980, 255.

51. **Changchien, L. M. and Craven, G. R.,** Studies on the role of amino acid residues 31 through 46 of ribosomal protein S4 in the mechanism of 30S ribosome assembly, *J. Mol. Biol.,* 125, 43, 1978.

52. **Funatsu, G., Puls, W., Schiltz, E., Reinholt, J., and Wittman, H. G.,** Ribosomal proteins XXXI. Comparative studies on altered proteins S4 of six *Escherichia coli* revertants from streptomycin dependence, *Mol. Gen. Genet.,* 115, 131, 1972.

53. **Olsson, M. O. and Isaksson, L. A.,** Analysis of *rpsD* mutations in *Escherichia coli.* I. Comparison of mutants with various alterations in ribosomal protein S4, *Mol. Gen. Genet.,* 169, 251, 1979.

54. **Olsson, M. O.,** Analysis of *rpsD* mutations in *Escherichia coli.* II. Physiology of some representative mutants, *Mol. Gen. Genet.,* 169, 259, 1979.

55. **Olsson, M. O. and Isaksson, L. A.,** Analysis of *rpsD* mutations in *Escherichia coli.* III. Effects of *rpsD* mutations on expression of some ribosomal-protein genes, *Mol. Gen. Genet.,* 169, 271, 1979.

56. **Dabbs, E.R.,** The ribosomal components responsible for kasugamycin dependence, and its suppression in a mutant of *Escherichia coli, Mol. Gen. Genet.,* 177, 271, 1980.

57. **Subramanian, A. R. and Dabbs, E. R.,** Functional studies on ribosomes lacking protein L1 from mutant *Escherichia coli, Eur. J. Biochem.,* 112, 425, 1980.

58. **Jinks-Robertson, S. and Nomura, M.,** Regulation of ribosomal protein synthesis in an *Escherichia coli* mutant missing ribosomal protein L1, *J. Bacteriol.,* 145, 1445, 1981.

59. **Stöffler, G., Hazenbank, R., and Dabbs, E.R.,** Expression of the L11-L1 operon in mutants of *Escherichia coli,* lacking the ribosomal proteins L1 or L11, *Mol. Gen. Genet.,* 181, 164, 1981.

60. **Isono, K., Cumberlidge, A. G., Isono, S., and Hirota, Y.,** Further temperature-sensitive mutants of *Escherichia coli* with altered ribosomal proteins, *Mol. Gen. Genet.,* 152, 239, 1977.

61. **Whittman, H. G., Stöffler, G., Geyl, D., and Bock, A.,** Alterations of ribosomal proteins in revertants of a valyl-tRNA synthetase mutant of *Escherichia coli, Mol. Gen. Genet.,* 141, 317, 1975.

62. **Gold, L., O'Farrell, P. Z., and Russel, M.,** Regulation of gene 32 expression during bacteriophage T4 infection of *Escherichia coli, J. Biol. Chem.,* 251, 7251, 1976.

63. **Lemaire, G., Gold, L., and Yarus, M.,** Autogenous translational repression of bacteriophage T4 gene 32 expression *in vitro, J. Mol. Biol.,* 126, 73, 1978.

64. **Woese, C. R., Magrum, L. J., Gupta, R., Siegel, R. B., Stahl, D. A., Kop, J., Crawford, N., Brosius, J., Gutell, R., Hogan, J. J., and Noller, H. F.,** Secondary structure model for bacterial 16S ribosomal RNA: phylogenetic, enzymatic and chemical evidence, *Nucleic Acids Res.,* 8, 2275, 1980.

65. **Möller, K., Zwieb, C., and Brimacombe, R.,** Identification of the oligonucleotide and oligopeptide involved in an RNA-protein crosslink induced by ultraviolet irradiation of *Escherichia coli* 30S ribosomal subunits, *J. Mol. Biol.,* 126, 489, 1980.

66. **Zwieb, C. and Brimacombe, R.,** RNA-protein crosslinking in *Escherichia coli* 30S ribosomal subunits: precise localization of the nucleotide in 16S RNA which is coupled to protein S7 by ultraviolet irradiation, *Nucleic Acids Res.,* 6, 1775, 1978.

67. **Post, L. E. and Nomura, M.,** DNA sequences from the *str* operon of *Escherichia coli, J. Biol. Chem,* 255, 4660, 1980.

68. **Ungewickell, E., Garrett, R., Ehresmann, C., Stiegler, P., and Fellner, P.,** An investigation of the 16S binding sites of ribosomal proteins S4, S8, S15 and S20 from *Escherichia coli, Eur. J. Biochem.,* 51, 165, 1975.

69. **Zimmerman, R. A., Mackie, G. A., Muto, A., Garrett, R. A., Ungewickell, E., Ehresmann, C., Stiegler, P., Ebel, J. P., and Fellner, P.,** Location and characteristics of ribosomal protein binding sites in the 16S RNA of *Escherichia coli, Nucleic Acids Res.,* 2, 279, 1975.

70. **Johnson, M., Christensen, T., and Fiil, N. P.,** personal communication.

71. **Jinks-Robertson, S. and Nomura, M.,** unpublished experiments.

Chapter 4

THE SINGLE-STRANDED DNA BINDING PROTEIN OF BACTERIOPHAGE T4

Daniel H. Doherty, Peter Gauss, and Larry Gold

TABLE OF CONTENTS

I. INTRODUCTION

T4 is a complex bacteriophage whose genome contains more than 140 genes.[1] During T4 infection of *Escherichia coli,* at least 15 phage-encoded proteins are involved, directly or indirectly, in replication of T4 DNA.[1,2] One of these proteins, encoded by gene 32, has been the subject of considerable genetic, biochemical, and structural study in the past 18 years. At present, some aspects of the role of this protein in DNA metabolism in T4-infected cells are fairly well understood. The product of gene 32 (gp32) has been shown to be involved in T4 DNA replication,[3,4] molecular and genetic recombination,[5-8] and the repair of ultraviolet light (UV) induced damage in T4 DNA.[9,10] Additionally, it has been shown that gp32 regulates its own synthesis.[11,12] Both in vivo[13] and in vitro[14] experiments indicate that gp32 specifically represses its own synthesis at the level of translation.

Over ten years ago, Alberts and Frey[15] showed that purified gp32 binds to single-stranded DNA (ssDNA) and that this binding is cooperative. It is now known that gp32 also binds unstructured RNA's, although at a much lower affinity.[16,17] This affinity for single-stranded nucleic acids could potentially explain the role of gp32 in replication, recombination, and repair. The protein might simply bind to and protect regions of ssDNA which are transiently produced during the processes of replication, recombination, and repair. This property could also explain autogenous translational control. Autogenous control of translation could be achieved after ssDNA is saturated, caused by the specific binding of gp32 to its own message.

Alternatively, the gene 32 protein might have a role in DNA replication beyond merely binding to single-stranded regions of DNA. Alberts[18] in 1974 proposed what he termed a "glamorous" model for gp32 action. He suggested that, in addition to binding ssDNA at the replication fork, gp32 might interact synergistically with the T4 DNA polymerase and facilitate the opening of double-stranded DNA in advance of the polymerase. These suggestions were made on the basis of experiments showing that gp32 could bind T4 DNA polymerase[19] and that gp32 could denature poly [d(A-T)].[15] An even more glamorous model has been proposed by Mosig. Based primarily on genetic studies by her and her collaborators she has proposed that gp32 has direct and specific interactions with no fewer than ten T4 proteins involved in T4 DNA replication and recombination.[20-22]

In this review, we hope to develop a picture of the in vivo role of gp32 in T4 DNA metabolism. We propose to do this through the following: (a) We will summarize the current understanding of gp32 binding to nucleic acids, attempting to relate functional domains of the protein to particular parameters of nucleic acid binding. A more detailed treatment of these topics can be found in Kowalczykowski et al.[23] and Williams and Konigsberg;[24] (b) We will describe the relevant in vivo and in vitro experiments which characterize the involvement of gp32 in T4 nucleic acid metabolism. We will stress the potential for the nucleic-acid binding properties of gp32, as described in Section II, to account for the observed effects of in vivo and in vitro manipulation of the protein. Specifically, we will evaluate the need to postulate a "glamorous" role for gp32 as opposed to the more limited or "passive" role of a single-stranded DNA binding protein; (c) We will critically examine the evidence for gp32 participation in specific protein-protein interactions with other T4 (and *E. coli*) proteins involved in T4 DNA metabolism. We will attempt to determine in which instances there is clear evidence for direct and specific protein-protein contacts as opposed to "interactions" which could easily be indirect; and (d) On the basis of the above, we will construct a model describing, on the basis of current evidence, the most probable in vivo role(s) of gp32 in T4 DNA metabolism.

II. FUNCTIONAL DOMAINS OF gp32 INVOLVED IN NUCLEIC ACID BINDING

A. Binding Properties of Intact gp32

In 1968, Alberts et al.[25] identified the protein product of gene 32. A protein that tightly bound single-stranded DNA (ssDNA) was absent from lysates of cells infected with a nonsense mutant of gene 32 and present in all other mutant infections tested. Using DNA-cellulose chromatography Alberts and Frey purified gp32.[15] The purified protein was found to bind tightly and cooperatively to ssDNA. Additionally, purified gp32 was shown to melt double-stranded poly[d(A-T)], shifting the Tm from 65°C to 25°C. However, double-stranded DNA (dsDNA) of T4 (or any other naturally occurring DNA) was not denatured by gp32. The protein was also found to increase the rate of renaturation of denatured DNA, presumably because ssDNA bound to gp32 is structurally altered. There is, in fact, direct evidence that ssDNA bound by gp32 is structurally altered. Phage fd ssDNA, when saturated with gp32, sediments only 1.3 times faster in sucrose gradients than does uncomplexed DNA, although the gp32-bound DNA complex has 13 times the mass of uncomplexed DNA.[15] Additionally, electron microscopy of bacteriophage ΦX174 ssDNA bound by gp32 reveals that the contour length of the bound DNA is about 50% greater than that of the uncomplexed form.[26]

The ideas that emerged from these early in vitro characterizations of the gene 32 protein were that:

1. gp32 might act in DNA replication in vivo by binding and protecting transiently single-stranded DNA sequences at the replication fork.
2. Given the ability of gp32 to denature poly [d(A-T)], the protein might act in vivo to denature locally duplex DNA in advance of DNA polymerase.
3. gp32 could promote recombination by holding ssDNA in an extended conformation, suitable for renaturation between complementary sequences.

Recently the binding of gp32 to short oligonucleotides (2 to 8 nucleotides in length) and longer polynucleotides has been examined in detail.[16] In characterizing the physical-chemical parameters of these interactions, distinct differences between the binding of gp32 to oligonucleotides and polynucleotides were observed. Binding to oligonucleotides is not cooperative, and is insensitive to salt concentration, base composition, sugar (ribose or deoxyribose), and the length (between 2 and 8) of the oligonucleotide. The observation that binding of gp32 to oligonucleotides was the same for lengths 2 through 8 suggests that in this mode of binding gp32 might be interacting with only 1 or 2 nucleotide residues, perhaps at an end. Such a binding mechanism ought to be different from the in vivo situation in which gp32 coats long stretches of ssDNA which lack ends. Newport et al.[17] examined the parameters of gp32 binding to long nucleic acids. Binding of gp32 to polynucleotides was found to be salt sensitive, and cooperative;[16] the cooperativity was not salt sensitive. Polynucleotides containing deoxyribose were the favored substrate over ribose-containing polynucleotides, and some binding specificity resulting from base composition was also demonstrated. In contrast, the cooperativity (which can be measured only in the polynucleotide mode) was virtually independent of sugar type or base composition. The preference of gp32 for deoxyribonucleotides in the polynucleotide mode is sufficiently great to ensure that, in vivo, ssDNA will be saturated prior to gp32 binding to any other nucleic acid species. Only after saturation of ssDNA will gp32 be available to bind unstructured regions of RNA.

B. Binding Properties of Proteolytic Fragments of gp32

Structural domains of proteins are portions of a polypeptide that can act autonomously; that is, they independently possess some property of an individual protein.[27] For example,

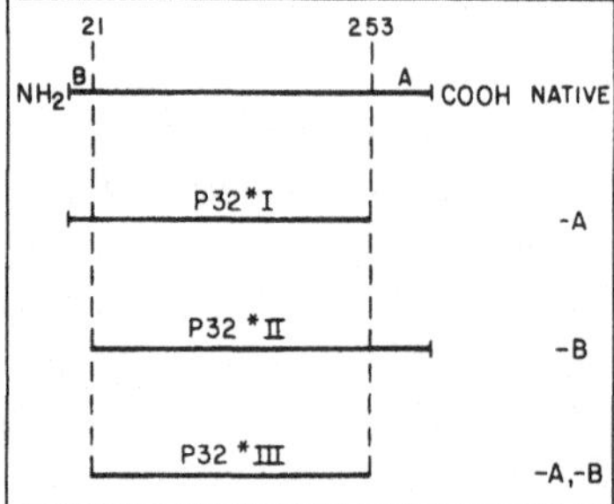

POLYPEPTIDE		BINDING TO DNA CELLULOSE						COOPERATIVITY		SALT SENSITIVITY		DENATURES ds DNA
		ss DNA			ds DNA							
		.05M NaCl	.4M NaCl	2.0M NaCl	.025M NaCl	.1M NaCl	.4M NaCl	OLIGO-NUCLEOTIDES	POLY-NUCLEOTIDES	OLIGO-NUCLEOTIDES	POLY-NUCLEOTIDES	
NATIVE		+	+	−	−	−	−	NO	YES	NO	YES	NO
P32*I −A		+	−	−	+	+	−	NO	YES	YES	YES	YES
P32*II −B		+	−	−	−	−	−	*	*	*	*	*
P32*III −A,−B		+	−	−	+	−	−	NO	NO	YES	YES	*

FIGURE 1.   This figure summarizes a large body of work describing the properties of proteolytic fragments of gp32. Simply stated, many lines of evidence converge to show that loss of the aminoterminal 21 residues of the protein (the B peptide) abolishes cooperative binding. Loss of the carboxyterminal 48 residues (the A peptide) confers the ability to denature double-stranded DNA. Loss of the A peptide also renders gp32 binding to oligonucleotides salt sensitive.

the cI repressor protein of bacteriophage lambda has been shown to contain two domains.[28] Partial proteolysis of cI protein yields two fragments, one containing the aminoterminus, the other containing the carboxyterminus. Each of these fragments independently possesses one function of the mature protein. The native protein binds to specific nucleotide sequences in λ DNA (the operators) and also forms dimers. The aminoterminal fragment binds operator DNA, but does not dimerize.[29] Conversely, the carboxyterminal fragment forms dimers but does not bind the operator sequences.[28]

The domains of gp32 considered below are not strictly analogous to the cI protein domains. Generally, gp32 domains have been identified by analysis of products of limited proteolysis. Loss of a particular function can be correlated to loss of a particular peptide. However, the "lost" function has not been demonstrated to reside autonomously in the lost peptide fragment. Domains thus defined might directly execute particular functions but might also affect such functions indirectly through contributions to the three dimensional structure of the protein.

Identification of functional domains in gp32 has centered around the analysis of three truncated polypeptides produced by limited proteolysis of native gp32. These products of partial proteolysis were first described by Moise and Hosoda.[30] Limited treatment of gp32 with any of three bovine proteases (trypsin, alpha-chymotrypsin, or pepsin) produced a mixture of peptides with estimated molecular weights of 27,000, 34,000, and 26,000 daltons. The molecular weight of intact gp32 is approximately 35,000. The three fragments were designated P32*I, P32*II, and P32*III respectively. P32*I is derived from native gp32 through loss of 48 amino acids (usually termed the A peptide) from the carboxyterminus.[31] P32*III also lacks the first 21 amino acids, termed the B peptide, at the aminoterminus of the protein, as well as the A peptide. By inference, the 34,000 dalton polypeptide (P32*II) lacks only the B peptide. Varied analyses[30-34] of the in vitro properties of these proteolytic fragments have presented a consistent picture of functional properties of gp32 associated with the presence or absence of the A and B peptides. These properties are described in Figure 1.

Elimination of the aminoterminal B peptide abolishes cooperative binding but has no affect on the intrinsic binding affinity. The elimination of the carboxyterminal A peptide seemingly allows gp32 to "bind" dsDNA. In fact, this apparent binding to dsDNA has been shown to arise through denaturation and binding to ssDNA.[35] P32*I has been shown to lower the Tm of T4 DNA by 50°C.[32] Loss of the A peptide thus allows gp32 to melt dsDNA. Native

(a) Oligonucleotide binding mode

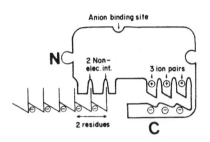

(b) Polynucleotide binding mode

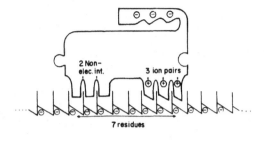

(c) Co-operative polynucleotide binding mode

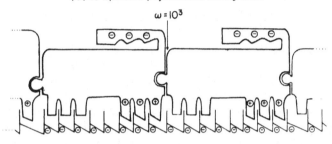

FIGURE 2. This figure, shows the model of von Hippel and collaborators for gp32 binding to nucleic acids. Binding to oligonucleotides (2a) does not utilize the salt sensitive binding site while binding to longer polynucleotides (2b) does. Utilization of the salt sensitive site involves displacement of the acidic carboxyterminus (C) from that site by the acidic phosphates of nucleic acids. Cooperative binding (2c) occurs only to polynucleotides but not to oligonucleotides. Cooperativity results from contacts between gp32 monomers. These contacts involve the aminoterminus (N). Cooperative binding results in a contiguous chain of bound gp32 molecules coating a stretch of nucleic acid. (From Kowalczykowski, S. C., Lonberg, N., Newport, J. W., and von Hippel, P. H., *J. Mol. Biol.*, 145, 75, 1981. With permission.)

gp32 does not lower the Tm of T4 DNA at all.[15] Loss of the A peptide has no affect on cooperativity, but slightly increases the intrinsic binding affinity; P32*I binds to oligonucleotides with a 2 to 3 times greater affinity than does native gp32.[33,34] Additionally, this binding is now salt sensitive, unlike the binding of native gp32 to oligonucleotides. Given that polynucleotide binding by unprocessed gp32 is salt sensitive and that the cooperativity evident in polynucleotide binding is not salt sensitive,[16] Lonberg et al.[34] have suggested that elimination of the A peptide makes a salt sensitive ligand interaction site on the protein more available, and thus increases the binding affinity. Normally, this salt sensitive site only interacts with ssDNA when binding occurs in the polynucleotide mode.

The model for gp32 binding to ssDNA that emerges from these studies is shown in Figure 2. In the model, the carboxyterminal A peptide blocks a salt sensitive DNA interaction site. Cooperative binding to polynucleotides utilizes this site by displacing the A peptide; binding to short oligonucleotides does not. Cooperativity is postulated to arise from protein-protein interactions involving the aminoterminal B peptide. Studies on protease sensititivity ofGP32 bound to oligo- and polynucleotides support this idea. Binding of gp32 to polynucleotides, but not oligonucleotides, decreases trypsin sensitivity of the B peptide cleavage and simultaneously increases the sensitivity of the A peptide cleavage.[31]

This blocking of the salt sensitive DNA binding site by the A peptide may explain the denaturation capacity of P32*I. The inability of native gp32 to melt dsDNA has been shown to arise from a "kinetic block" which prevents gp32 from nucleating transiently open regions of duplex DNA.[36] Spicer et al.[33] propose that the acquired ability of P32*I, which lacks the A peptide, to overcome this block, results from a faster forward rate constant or, "on rate" for ssDNA binding. This notion remains to be tested, but it seems unlikely that the small increase in binding affinity for ssDNA exhibited by P32*I accounts entirely for the ability of this peptide to melt duplex DNA.[33,36]

In summary, these in vitro binding studies indicate that the core of gp32, i.e., P32*III, which lacks the aminoterminal B peptide and the carboxyterminal A peptide, retains most of the information for contacting ssDNA. However, P32*III has lost the ability to interact with other molecules of gp32 in a manner that brings about cooperative binding. Loss of cooperative binding is correlated with the absence of the B peptide. Additionally, the core peptide denatures dsDNA due to the absence of the carboxyterminal A peptide.

C. Amino Acid Sequences of the A and B Peptides

The amino acid sequence of gp32 is known,[37] as are the protease-sensitive sites which give rise to P32*I and P32*III, when gp32 is cleaved.[31] Therefore, one can examine the amino acid sequences of the A and B peptides. The aminoterminal B peptide is thought to be largely alpha-helical (based on secondary structure predictions of Williams and Konigsberg[31]) and contains five (out of a total of 21) positively charged residues, including three contiguous basic residues (lys-arg-lys at positions 3 through 5). However, given the insensitivity of cooperativity to salt concentration,[16] the loss of cooperative binding associated with loss of the B peptide cannot result from elimination of electrostatic interactions that utilize these basic residues. Again, we note that the B peptide may not directly interact with other gp32 molecules. Rather, the evidence to date proves only that loss of the B peptide affects the interaction of gp32 proteins. This effect could be indirect.

The sequence of the A peptide is unusual in several respects. Out of a total of 48 residues, this peptide contains 14 acidic groups; 6 of the terminal 12 residues are aspartic acid. A cluster of serine residues, comprising 8 of 9 residues, is found at positions 280 to 288. The predicted secondary structure[37] is about equally divided between alpha-helix and random coil. It is not clear how any of these features of the sequence relate to the in vivo function of this region, although the presence of clustered acidic residues at the carboxyterminus of gp32 may be significant. A similar cluster of acidic residues is found at the carboxyterminal end of the ssDNA binding protein of *E. coli*.[38] The carboxyterminal 12 residues of this protein contain 5 acidic groups. Similarly, the carboxyterminus of the ssDNA binding protein of bacteriophage T7 (which is unrelated to T4) is negatively charged; twelve of the terminal 16 residues are acidic.[39] A possible role for the negatively charged A peptide of the T4 protein has been suggested[34] (see Figure 2); this region might be involved in electrostatic blockage of the salt sensitive binding site utilized in the polynucleotide binding mode, but not in the oligonucleotide binding mode. In the absence of ssDNA, the carboxyterminus might interact with basic residues at the DNA binding site.

D. Genetic Evidence for Domains

Temperature sensitive and amber mutations in gene 32 have been isolated by several laboratories.[3,40] However, the number of gene 32 mutations in the classic collections of T4 mutants is small [4 temperature sensitive (*ts*), 3 amber, and one UGA] and the positions of the mutations are in the aminoterminal half of the protein molecule. The temperature sensitive mutations map within the first one-third of the protein.[40] The clustering of gene 32 mutations has been interpreted by Mosig et al.[22] and Breschkin and Mosig[41] to indicate that all residues essential for DNA replication are aminoterminal to the amber mutation amA453. In addition, Breschkin and Mosig[41] suggest that the amber peptides retain all functions necessary for one round of T4 DNA replication, and that even the shortest amber fragment (from A453) can still bind to ssDNA.[22] However, a host function, as yet unidentified, could be substituting for gp32 in the amber mutant infections. One round of DNA replication might be driven by the host protein rather than the A453 amber fragment. Additionally, some of the temperature

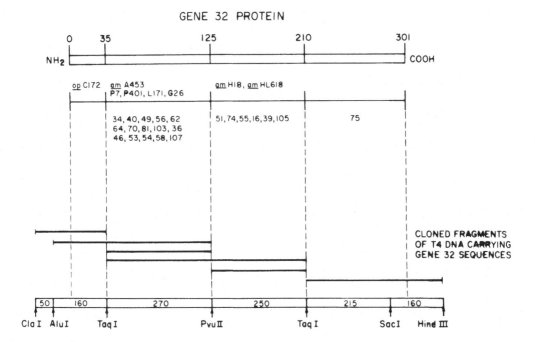

FIGURE 3. We have cloned a series of restriction fragments that include all, or portions of, the gene 32 coding sequence. Some of these fragments, and a partial restriction map of this region are shown here. We have mapped our newly isolated gene 32 mutations, and the classical mutations, to various cloned restriction fragments. The map thus derived is shown above. Using the partial DNA sequence of gene 32[76] and the nucleotide sequence information inherent in the amino acid sequence of Williams et al.,[37] we have aligned our restriction map to the amino acid sequence of gp32 and identified the positions in the protein that correspond to restriction fragment endpoints in the gene. Therefore, we can localize the positions of amino acid alterations to defined segments of the protein. Classical mutations are shown above the line, and our newly isolated missense mutations shown below. Each number represents a recombinationally distinct site.

sensitive mutants show less DNA synthesis than do the amber mutations, and this is difficult to understand. Although one idea is that the *ts* mutations directly wreck DNA binding, another interpretation would have a nonfunctional missense mutant protein prevent substitution by the substituting host function. Finally, the original number of mutations available in gene 32 is too small to see domains as separable genetic targets. This latter point prevents a unique interpretation of the clustering of the classical gene 32 mutations.

Recently, we have undertaken an extensive mutant hunt using a special host[42] to identify missense mutations in gene 32. Using hydroxylamine, we have mutagenized T4 extensively and isolated over 100 temperature sensitive mutations in gene 32 (see Figure 3). We now know that many essential amino acid residues are present carboxyterminal to the site of amber A453. Missense mutations are not restricted to the aminoterminus; we have isolated at least one mutation that maps in the distal one-third of the protein. These mutations have been localized to particular restriction fragments by marker rescue experiments from cloned fragments of T4 DNA that contain portions of the gene 32 coding sequence. A map of these mutations is shown in Figure 3.

Our preliminary findings have led us to conclude that the genetic map of gene 32 of Mosig et al.[40,41] is an incomplete representation of the essential sites within the protein. We find a distinct clustering of temperature sensitive mutations in the promoter proximal portion of the gene (i.e., between residues 35 and 125); however a number of *ts* mutations are found between residues 125 and 210. There is a corresponding paucity of mutations in the extreme aminoterminal and carboxyterminal regions of the gene 32 protein. Preliminary results have shown that all the mutations thus far tested (including *ts* 75, the most carboxyterminal mutation) affect DNA replication to some extent.

E. A Putative Binding Site for ssDNA

On the basis of secondary structure predictions, Williams et al.[37] suggested that gp32 could be divided into 3 domains. The aminoterminal region (residues 1 to 35) and the carboxyterminal region (residues 187 to 301) are each primarily alpha-helical. The central region of the protein (residues 36 to 186) contains most of the beta sheet structures and beta turns. These investigators pointed out some interesting features of the region around residues 72 through 116. This region contains 6 of the 8 tyrosine residues found in the protein and 5 of these are nearly equally spaced in the primary structure. This region is predicted to be composed of three- short beta sheets separated by beta turns. This predicted secondary structure is similar to the actual structure of the DNA binding site of the ssDNA binding protein of bacteriophage fd. As determined by X-ray crystallography at 2.3 A resolution, the bulk of the amino acid residues that interact with ssDNA reside in a three-stranded beta structure comprised of about 40 residues.[43] This beta structure contains several aromatic residues which could interact with bound DNA by intercalation. Indeed, in the case of the fd ssDNA binding protein, tyrosine intercalation is known to be involved in DNA binding.[44,45] In the case of gp32, there is also some indication that tyrosine intercalation may be involved in DNA binding.[46]

It is interesting to note that our newly isolated mutations in gene 32 are clustered near, or in, this very region. We found no mutations which map between residues 1 and 35 and only one which maps carboxyterminal to residue 210. In contrast, we found 21 mutational sites between residues 35 and 210. Of these, 6 are between residues 126 and 210 while 15 map between 36 and 125. We have also shown that the four previously known *ts* alleles of gene 32 map between residues 36 and 125. We are currently investigating the distribution of mutations within the region between residues 36 and 125, and the distribution of sites between 126 and 205. More detailed localization of these mutations coupled with in vivo and in vitro characterization of defective proteins should help to delineate functional domains of the protein.

In summary, based on the protein sequence, chemical modification experiments, genetic studies, and an analogy to another ssDNA binding protein, we suggest that the region including residues 72 through 116 may be involved directly in ssDNA binding. Proof of this hypothesis will await crystallographic solution of gp32 and/or detailed cross-linking studies.

III. GENE 32 FUNCTION IN VIVO AND IN VITRO DURING NUCLEIC ACID METABOLISM

A. In Vivo Roles of Gene 32 Protein During DNA Metabolism

In vivo the gene 32 protein is essential for DNA replication, recombination and repair. We will briefly review the experiments that suggest this involvement.

1. DNA Synthesis

The work of Epstein et al.[3] first suggested that gene 32 mutant infections were defective in DNA synthesis. Subsequent experiments were directed at determining the fate of parental and newly synthesized DNA after infections with gene 32 amber mutants. These experiments involved the use of density labeled parental phage DNA. DNA synthesis was measured as the production of hybrid or light density DNA after infection with heavy labeled phage. These molecules can be distinguished by their banding pattern in cesium chloride density gradients. Using these techniques, Kozinski and Felgenhauer[7] showed that gene 32 mutant infections do produce hybrid DNA molecules and therefore proceed through at least one round of replication. However, no fully light DNA is produced, indicating that no additional rounds of replication occur. The parental DNA molecules are extensively degraded to small fragments and eventually to acid-soluble material. Additional experiments showed a decrease in the amount of single-stranded DNA in gene 32 mutant infections compared to wild type infections. These results for the first time suggested that the gene 32 protein might be involved in the protection of single-stranded DNA.

The gene 32 protein is continuously required for DNA synthesis. Riva et al.[4] and Curtiss and Alberts[47] found that infections with gene 32 mutant *ts* P7 showed an "immediate stop" phenotype if the infected cells were shifted from low to high temperature at a time after DNA synthesis had already begun. Curtiss and Alberts suggested that the immediate stop phenotype for this mutant infection resulted from the involvement of the mutant gene product in reactions at active replication forks.[47]

During DNA synthesis in vivo, the proteins associated with the replication complex, including gp32, have an additional role in assuring the fidelity of the polymerization reaction.[48,49] In vitro the presence of these proteins in the replication reaction increases fidelity approximately 100-fold.[50] It has not yet been determined how these proteins affect error rates. One could speculate either that the accessory proteins directly interact with polymerase to affect nucleotide selection or that these proteins alter the DNA template to permit a more exacting examination of DNA by DNA polymerase. The answer to this question awaits further in vitro experimentation.

2. Recombination

Physical measurement of recombination between parental molecules requires that one parental phage be density labeled (e.g., with C^{13} and N^{15}). These phage are then used to coinfect cells with light (i.e., C^{12} and N^{13}) phage. The cells are infected in light media, and the conditions are chosen to prevent phage DNA replication. The production of hybrid density phage DNA is only possible via recombination. Two types of hybrid DNA have been identified after infection with wild type phage. The first type is termed a joint recombinant molecule. This hybrid molecule has a noncovalent recombinant structure that is stabilized only by hydrogen bonds and is a putative intermediate to the second class of hybrid, a true covalent recombinant molecule. Joint molecules can be resolved into fully heavy and fully light components after denaturation and CsCl centrifugation. To become a covalent recombinant molecule that is stable to denaturation, the joint molecule must be acted upon by DNA ligase and/or DNA polymerase. Tomizawa et al.[5] studied the formation of T4 joint recombinant DNA molecules after infection with heavy and light density labelled parental phage. After T4 gene 32 mutant infections, no joint recombinant molecules were observed. As we have already noted, Kozinski and Felgenhauer[7] found that gene 32 mutant infections were also deficient in the amount of single-stranded DNA present after infection. They suggested that single-stranded DNA was required for recombination and that the major role of gp32 was to permit the accumulation of single-stranded DNA during T4 infection. Genetic studies by Berger et al.[8] and Mosig et al.[40] indicated that gene 32 mutations decreased the frequency of recombination between two closely linked rII mutations. Finally, Broker and Lehman[6] and Broker[51] showed that gp32 was essential for the formation of branched recombinational intermediates (viewed in the electron microscope) after T4 infection. Gene 32 mutant infections resulted in a ten-fold decrease in the number of branched recombination intermediates observed. These branched structures could correspond to either type of hybrid DNA, that is, joint or covalent recombinant molecules. The suggestion was made that gp32 may protect single-stranded DNA from nuclease digestion and also facilitate pairing of homologous DNA molecules by extending the single strands into an appropriate configuration.

3. Repair

Experiments by Baldy[9] first suggested that gp32 may be involved in the repair of UV damaged T4 phage. These experiments measured the kinetics of phage inactivation by UV irradiation and indicated that phage with the temperature sensitive mutation *ts* L171 in gene 32 were more sensitive to irradiation than wild type phage. Further examination of the role of gp32 in the repair of UV damage by Wu and Yeh[10] suggested that gp32 was essential for the maintenance of unit length T4 DNA molecules after UV irradiation of T4 infected cells. Even in the absence of DNA damage, gp32 is required for DNA integrity. Curtiss and Alberts[47] showed that temperature shift-up (to 42°) after infection with the gene 32 mutant *ts* P7 not only stopped DNA synthesis, but resulted in degradation of the replicated DNA by an endonuclease encoded by T4. In the next section we will review in vitro experiments that suggest the involvement of gp32 in the protection of single-stranded DNA from nuclease digestion. Perhaps low levels of gp32 activity during gene 32 mutant infections result in increases susceptability of single-stranded DNA to nucleases. Nuclease cuts in these single-stranded DNA regions probably can not be repaired.

These experiments confirm the important in vivo roles of gene 32 protein in replication, recombination and repair. *The phenotypes of 32⁻ infections could all result from the failure to protect single-stranded DNA from nuclease digestion and/or the failure to provide an extended configuration for cellular ssDNA.* The phenotypes themselves do not demand a glamorous model.

B. In Vitro Roles of gp32 During DNA Synthesis

Continuous DNA replication in vivo after T4 infection requires at least 16 different T4 gene products (for review see Broker and Doermann[2]). However, only gene products 32, 41, 43, 44, 45, 61, and 62 are needed for in vitro DNA replication of a nicked double-stranded DNA template. These proteins are necessary and sufficient for both leading and lagging-strand DNA synthesis at a replication fork as summarized in Figure 4. (This is summarized from the work of Alberts and collaborators, see Liu et al.[50] See also Silver and Nossal[52]). The known activities of these gene products in vitro are summarized in Table 1. Our purpose in this section is to examine the role of gp32 in this replication complex.

1. gp32 Alone

One function of gp32 at the replication fork may be to alter single-stranded DNA such that it acts as an efficient template for DNA polymerization. Many experiments have suggested that the binding of gp32 changes the structure of single-stranded DNA (see Section II.A, above). Besides these early measurements, we now know that gp32 increases the UV adsorption of ssDNA and also alters its ultraviolet circular dichroism.[36,46,53] These changes in DNA structure may cause the increased rate of renaturation of denatured DNA when gp32 is present. By extending the DNA backbone and leaving the bases exposed for pairing with complementary single-stranded DNA, the first and rate limiting nucleation step of renaturation becomes more efficient. The gene 32 protein increases the rate of T4 DNA renaturation 1000-fold.[15] In contrast to this, gp32 will stimulate denaturation of synthetic poly[d(A-T)] under conditions where the intramolecular duplex is stable.[15] This reaction is slower at higher magnesium ion concentrations, perhaps reflecting the increased competition of the renaturation reaction. The ability of gp32 to denature this polymer suggests the presence of transiently single-stranded regions sufficiently long for productive nucleation events that result in contiguous (cooperative) gp32 binding prior to complete renaturation.[36] Native T4 DNA does not contain such long single-stranded regions and is stable in the presence of gp32.[15,36] Thus, the inability of gp32 to denature double-stranded DNA is the result of a kinetic rather than thermodynamic block (see Section II.B and Jensen et al.[36]).

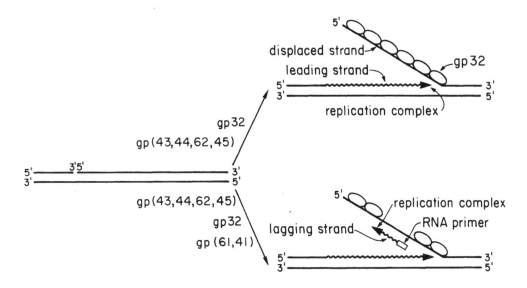

FIGURE 4. T4 DNA synthesis in vitro initiates at nicks in double-stranded DNA template molecules. The 3′ hydroxyl end at the site of the nick is used by the DNA polymerase (gp43) as a primer to initiate polymerization. As synthesis occurs, the 5′ side of the nicked molecule is displaced. The products of genes 43, 44, 45 and 62 (the replication complex) and gp32 are required for this reaction, termed leading strand synthesis. These proteins can not synthesize DNA de novo on single-stranded DNA; thus, there is no DNA synthesis on the displaced strand. When the products of genes 41 and 61 (RNA primase) are added to the above reaction, RNA oligomers are synthesized de novo on the single-stranded displaced strand. These oligomers are used as primers for DNA synthesis on the displaced strand. DNA synthesis occurring on the displaced strand is referred to as lagging strand synthesis.

Table 1
ACTIVITIES OF THE PROTEINS OF THE IN VITRO T4 DNA REPLICATION COMPLEX[a]

Genes	Proteins	Activities
43	DNA polymerase	Polymerization of dXTP's
32	ssDNA binding protein	Cooperative binding to ssDNA
44, 62, 45	Polymerase accessory protein	Enhancement of DNA polymerase processivity
41, 61	RNA primase	Synthesis of RNA primers

[a] Summarized from Liu et al.[50]

The binding of gene 32 protein to single-stranded DNA in vitro protects the bound polynucleotide from the action of several nucleases: the 3′ to 5′ exonuclease associated with the T4 DNA polymerase,[54] neurospora and S1 nuclease,[55] pancreatic DNase I,[47] and the recBC nuclease.[56] This protection probably reflects the in vivo requirement for gp32 in the accumulation of single-stranded DNA intermediates. This conclusion is supported by the in vivo results of Curtiss and Alberts[47] (noted in Section III.A) that suggest that gp32 is required for the integrity of concatemeric replicative intermediates. The most likely mechanism for gp32 protection of single-stranded DNA against nucleases is by occlusion of sensitive phosphodiester bonds. Once gp32 is bound to the polynucleotide, the potential of some proteins (in this case, nucleases) to interact with the DNA is diminished.

2. gp32 With Other Proteins of the T4 DNA Replication Complex
Any discussion of replication should distinguish between leading and lagging strand

synthesis (see Figure 4). To a first approximation lagging strand synthesis demands utilization and displacement of gp32 concomitant with DNA synthesis, whereas leading strand synthesis demands displacement of DNA. Strand displacement during leading strand synthesis provides potential binding sites for gp32 and, ultimately, the template upon which lagging strand synthesis occurs. Lagging strand synthesis (at least subsequent to primer synthesis) appears less complicated than leading strand synthesis; hence we discuss lagging strand synthesis first. The emphasis here is on the role of gp32 in each type of reaction. Additionally, we note that leading and lagging strand synthesis may occur in concert, due to the peculiar geometry of the replication apparatus.[57] Such conceptualization does not noticeably alter this discussion, since our focus is on gp32.

We first note the effect of gp32 on a simple replication system that uses partially single-stranded lambda DNA (generated by exoIII digestion) as template and only one other protein of the T4 replication system, DNA polymerase.[19] In this system (which mimics lagging-strand synthesis), gp32 stimulated DNA synthesis by the T4 DNA polymerase five to ten fold. Stimulation was greatest at low temperature and/or high salt concentration, conditions that favor intramolecular secondary structure in the template. The stimulation was interpreted as resulting from the removal of secondary structures present in the DNA template. However, denaturation of intramolecular structures is not sufficient to stimulate heterologous polymerases. The T4 single-stranded DNA binding protein does not stimulate *E. coli* DNA polymerase II but the *E. coli* single-stranded DNA binding protein (ssb gene product) does.[58] This suggests that each DNA polymerase prefers single-stranded DNA with a conformation imposed by its homologous single-stranded DNA binding protein. The different contour lengths for DNA-protein bound complexes with gp32 and ssb (4.6A/nucleotide[26] compared to 1.8A/nucleotide[58]) might reflect the base distortion required by the homologous polymerases for maximal stimulation of DNA synthesis in vitro (and perhaps in vivo). These results might also suggest that the stimulation of homologous polymerases is the result of direct protein-protein interactions between polymerase and single-stranded DNA binding protein. Such an interaction has been observed between gp32 and T4 DNA polymerase[19,59] (and see below). However, we note that protein-protein complexes have not been observed betwen the T7 DNA polymerase and T7 DNA binding protein.[60]

Stimulation of DNA synthesis by gp32 has also been examined using the synthetic polymer poly[d(A-T)] as template. This polymer is self-complementary and contains both linear, duplex, and hairpin structures.[61] Therefore, this template is intermediate between single-stranded and double-stranded DNA. Gene 32 protein stimulated DNA synthesis by T4 DNA polymerase approximately four fold with poly[d(A-T)] as template. This stimulation is probably due to the removal of secondary structures in poly[d(A-T)].[62] Using this system Gillan and Nossal[62] have studied the contributions of gp32 and gp43 to helix opening. This problem was approached by measuring DNA synthesis directed by mutant and wild type polymerases on the poly[d(A-T)] template. The results indicated that a mutant polymerase isolated from the DNA polymerase mutant *ts* CB120 incorporates labeled DNA precursors at a rate 30-fold less than wild type. The mutant enzyme does bind to the template. If gp32 is added to the reaction with *ts* CB120 polymerase, incorporation is stimulated 30-fold. In the reaction with wild type polymerase, the polymerase reaction is stimulated only four fold. These results could suggest that the *ts* CB120 polymerase is defective in translating the energy of hydrolysis of dXTP's to denaturation in front of the polymerase (see below). The deficiency of the *ts* CB120 polymerase is suppressed in the presence of gp32, perhaps by the ability of DNA binding protein to contribute to the rate of strand displacement.

Lagging strand synthesis can be studied in systems that utilize additional T4 proteins. A five protein replication system can use preprimed single-stranded DNA (like ϕX174) as a template. The five protein system includes the products of genes 32, 43, 44, 45, and 62. Several groups have reported that T4 DNA polymerase is stimulated by these other gene

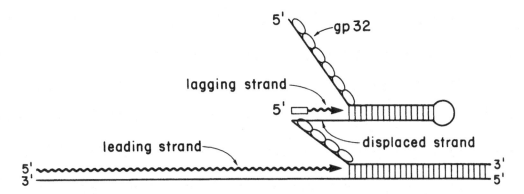

FIGURE 5. If hairpin structures can form on the displaced strand, the synthesis of the lagging strand requires the opening of duplex DNA in advance of the polymerase. As the stability of such hairpins increases, the requirements for lagging strand elongation become similar to those for elongation of the leading strand. Specifically, synthesis of lagging strand through a stable hairpin appears formally equivalent to leading strand synthesis through fully duplex DNA. Here we have drawn a slight distortion of the conventional representation of the replication fork in order to emphasize this potential equivalency of leading and lagging-strand synthesis.

products to increase the rate of DNA polymerization and increase as well the processivity of the DNA replication complex.[50,52,57,63-67] Some of the proteins in the replication complex may act to prevent the dissociation of DNA polymerase from the DNA template.[65,67] The hydrolysis of ATP may be required for this reaction. Recent results suggest that this replication complex, in the presence of the ATP analogue ATP-γ-S, will not proceed through double-stranded DNA regions but is still capable of replicating single-stranded DNA.[67] Most importantly, in the absence of the 32 protein or the 44, 45 and 62 proteins, DNA synthesis by DNA polymerase terminates at stable hairpin structures.[66,67] The presence of gp32 or a mixture of gp44, gp45, and gp62 enhanced DNA synthesis through these regions. Interestingly, the addition of all four proteins to the same reaction is synergystically stimulatory.

For DNA synthesis to occur *de novo* on single-stranded DNA, two additional proteins must be added to the previously described five protein system. These proteins are the products of genes 41 and 61, which by themselves are capable of synthesizing an oligoribonucleotide on single-stranded DNA.[50,64] This RNA molecule is utilized as a primer by DNA polymerase for the synthesis of DNA. This reaction models events that occur on the lagging strand when *de novo* synthesis is required but is similar in other respects to the five protein system discussed above. The important lesson from these cell free experiments is that gp32 does stimulate DNA synthesis on a single-stranded template. The stimulation derives from more than denaturation of the template strand, since other single-stranded binding proteins do not stimulate the T4 DNA polymerase. When the template DNA is structured (and especially when the T4 DNA polymerase, because of a mutation, does not do very well at replication on a structured template), gp32 stimulates DNA synthesis dramatically. When a stable hairpin is encountered, template denaturation and successful replication requires gp32 as well as the three other replication complex proteins. Most importantly, we note that replication through a stable hairpin on the single-stranded template bears topological similarity to the situation that occurs during leading strand synthesis (Figure 5); during such reactions gp32 is very important. Replication through a hairpin sets the stage for a discussion of leading strand synthesis.

Double-stranded DNA presents new problems during in vitro replication. T4 DNA polymerase alone cannot utilize nicked duplex T7 DNA as a template.[68] However, when gp32 is added to the reaction, a small amount of DNA is synthesized. Synthesis occurs only in low salt and in the presence of Mg^{++}; these conditions tend to destabilize AT rich regions

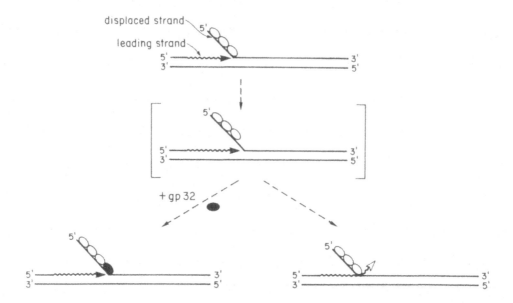

FIGURE 6.   Gene 32 protein may stimulate strand displacement synthesis simply by binding and stabilizing the single-stranded displaced strand. We propose the existence of an intermediate of the strand displacement reaction in which leading strand synthesis displaces a short stretch of ssDNA which is unbound by gp32. In the presence of gp32, the displaced, single-stranded, DNA is bound and stabilized. In the absence of gp32, the displaced strand can renature to the template strand, resulting in displacement of the leading strand and possibly of some of the replication complex proteins (denoted by an empty arrowhead). We note here (and in more detail in the text) that this model for stimulation of strand displacement synthesis is analogous to the mechanism by which single-stranded DNA binding proteins stabilize the ssDNA produced by the *helicase* activity of the recBC enzyme of *E. coli.*

of duplex DNA.[68] The DNA that is synthesized reflects the fact that AT-rich sequences are used as the template. The structure of the replicated molecules as visualized in the electron microscope also indicates that replication is proceeding aberrantly from random nicks that provide primers. The newly synthesized molecules have highly branched structures emanating from linear T7 molecules. In studies utilizing the same native T7 DNA as template, the gene 43 mutant *ts* CB120 polypeptide fails to polymerize DNA even in the presence of gp32.[62] Again, the *ts* CB120 polymerase binds to the DNA template; however, no stable incorporation occurs. This result suggests that gp32 and gp43 each have a role in strand displacement, and that the *ts* CB120 mutant peptide is defective in this activity.

For efficient in vitro DNA synthesis using nicked double-stranded DNA as template (i.e., replication of an entire molecule at nearly in vivo rates), the products of genes 44, 45, and 62 must be added to the gp43 plus gp32 reaction. The gene 32 protein is essential in this reaction; in its absence the DNA synthesis is reduced approximately 100-fold.[50,52] This suggests again that gp32 is required for the strand displacement reaction. This interpretation is supported by the experiments that show gp32 is not required for the first round of φX174 single-stranded DNA replication[50,52] (which involves copying of a single-stranded template) but is absolutely required for subsequent replication rounds after the template becomes double-stranded. The role of gp32 in strand displacement may be nothing more than facilitation of helix destabilization derived from binding to a short single-stranded intermediate (the displaced strand) produced by polymerase (Figure 6). That is, DNA polymerase may have the capacity to displace the equivalent of a gp32 monomer binding site, but no more. The facilitation does not, in itself, demand either a "glamorous" model or direct participation of gp32 in the strand displacement event.

This postulated stabilization of single-stranded DNA during replication is similar to the reactions observed when the recBC protein is incubated in vitro with double-stranded DNA + ATP.[56,69] During this incubation, single-stranded DNA (the substrate for recombination) is generated by the helicase activity of the recBC protein working from one end of the double-stranded DNA. This single-stranded DNA has two possible fates. In the presence of gp32[56] or ssb,[69] the displaced strands remain single-stranded and are protected from the nuclease activity associated with the recBC protein; in the absence of ssb or gp32, the single-stranded DNA is eventually renatured or, under conditions that activate the nuclease activity, degraded. This reaction is analogous to the strand displacement reaction at a replication fork as diagrammed in Figure 6. The recBC protein and the replication complex produce single-stranded DNA, the substrate for gp32 in vivo and in vitro. This single-stranded DNA is stable *only in the presence of gp32*. The gene 32 protein (or ssb) plays no role in the unwinding reactions of either protein complex; yet, its presence is essential for the stable production of single-stranded DNA. In vivo, the ssb-complexed (bound) ssDNA generated by the recBC reaction becomes the substrate for recombination; the gp32-bound ssDNA generated by the strand displacement reaction (Figure 6) usually becomes the template for the synthesis of the lagging strand.

In summary, total DNA synthesis using nicked double-stranded DNA molecules as templates requires the seven protein system. These replication proteins polymerize nucleotides into DNA using a DNA or RNA primer, displace the complementary DNA strand, move the polymerase along the template, and initiate the synthesis of RNA primers on the displaced strand. None of these reactions occur in the absence of gp32. The entire nature of this requirement is still undetermined; however, it is clear that only the presence of gp32 enables polymerase and accessory proteins to replicate templates with extensive secondary structure. Since neither gp32 nor the other individual proteins of the replication complex denature native DNA, we assume that the complex association of proteins at a replication fork provides additional sites on the DNA and sources of energy that facilitate helix melting and strand displacement. We may also have suggested that *homologous* DNA binding proteins are more important for lagging strand synthesis than for leading strand synthesis. We are unaware of any data that precisely answer this question.

C. Autogenous Translational Regulation of gp32 Expression (an Aside)

During the late 1960s and early 1970s biologists concerned with T4 development began to examine the global pattern of T4 gene expression. Specific T4 gene products were identified after examination of the proteins expressed when the infecting phage was mutant in a particular gene.[70,71] Most T4 gene products are regulated transcriptionally using temporally differentiated recognition of at least three classes of promoters.[72,73] Gene 32 expression was found to be regulated by a unique system.[11-13] Two elements were found that regulate the synthesis of gp32; the level of ssDNA present and the gene 32 protein itself. Any T4 infection that diminished the level of intracellular single-stranded T4 DNA showed diminished levels of gene 32 expression; infected cells that contained high levels of single-stranded DNA showed enhanced levels of gene 32 expression. Independent of the level of single-stranded DNA, cells infected by gene 32 mutants always overproduced the aberrant gene 32 product. Even gene 32 missense mutants, *under permissive conditions,* showed overproduction of the mutant protein. In such experiments the only difference between a mutant infection and a wild type infection was the quality (and quantity) of the gene 32 product; the kinetics of DNA synthesis were identical in the two infections. These results were used to generate a model for gene 32 expression:[11,13] single-stranded DNA was established as an inducer of gp32 expression, and the gene 32 protein was defined as a repressor of gene 32 expression. Although the notion of autogenous, negative regulation had been described as a formal possibility,[74] the gene 32 regulatory system was the first example for which the data were convincing. In the regulatory model, the primary target for gene 32 protein was single-stranded DNA; when all available single-stranded DNA was titrated, the accumulation of more gene 32 protein led to repression of further expression.

The regulatory system was further dissected by both in vivo[13] and in vitro[14] experiments. Regulation was found to occur at the level of translation. The gene 32 mRNA was found to be completely stable, repression and derepression were reversible (in vivo and in vitro), derepression could be obtained without any transcription, and cells fully repressed for gene 32 expression contained large quantities of gene 32 mRNA that was efficiently translated in vitro.[13] The gene 32 protein was found to behave as a specific inhibitor of gene 32 translation.[14] Even induction of gene 32 expression by single-stranded DNA was demonstrated in vitro; incubations containing gene 32 protein at concentrations sufficient for repression of gene 32 expression could be titrated with single-stranded DNA so as to allow translation at the depressed level.

These experiments were entirely consistent with the detailed model for autogenous translational repression proposed by Gold et al.[11] and Russell et al.[13] The data did not (and still does not) demand that the target for repression is the gene 32 mRNA; a formal possibility remains that the repressor binds to ribosomes and thereby alters the translational specificity of those ribosomes. However, the model, in attempting to utilize known qualities of gene 32 protein, ignored that formal possibility. The model (Figure 7) proposed that the gene 32 mRNA contained a uniquely unstructured domain surrounding the initiation codon, and that repression came about via cooperative binding of gp32 to this domain. The unstructured domain was postulated to include (in the model) nucleotides 3′ to the initiation codon, since ribosome binding sites (see Gold et al.[75]) certainly include nucleotides from the aminoterminal coding portion of the gene. Lemaire et al.[14] also suggested that the unstructured domain coevolved with the aminoterminal residues of gp32, changing both the site of repression (the translational operator) and the repressor activity of the gene 32 protein.

Krisch et al.[76] have presented a short DNA sequence from the region of gene 32 containing the proposed operator (Figure 7). The very region proposed as the gp32 binding site is more unstructured than any other sequence of equivalent length yet obtained in T4.[77] Furthermore, the unstructured domain does extend 3′ to the initiation codon, allowing one to imagine that coevolution as proposed by Lemaire et al.[14] might have occurred. The operator, as an unstructured domain, is long enough to bind several monomers of gp32, just as shown in the original model. For an unstructured domain of this size, extreme cooperativity of binding would be essential for gp32 to fill this domain rather than to scatter onto many slightly shorter unstructured RNA domains present in every mRNA. Specific repression, in this model, is a function of the cooperativity of gene 32 binding to nucleic acid ligands. In fact, the large cooperativity intrinsic to the gene 32 protein is derived (at least in part) from the aminoterminus of the protein. Cooperativity is obliterated when the aminoterminal residues are removed proteolytically.[34] The residues of gp32 that contribute to cooperativity are encoded by the highly nonrandom, unstructured domain that, we think, comprise the operator.

A lengthy discussion of the uniqueness of this particular nucleotide sequence in gene 32 and the role of cooperativity in the prior filling of single-stranded DNA and the specificity of repression has been presented elsewhere;[77] the ideas are mentioned here merely to demonstrate that even the autogenous translational repression of gene 32 expression could utilize nothing more than the known and simple qualities of gene 32 protein: (1) an affinity for single-stranded nucleic acids; (2) tighter binding to DNA than RNA; and (3) highly cooperative binding to nucleic acids. Thus, even the glamorous function of translational repression may occur without glamorous biochemistry.

IV. EVIDENCE FOR SPECIFIC INTERACTIONS BETWEEN gp32 AND OTHER REPLICATION PROTEINS

In the previous section, we emphasized the potential of the known binding affinity of

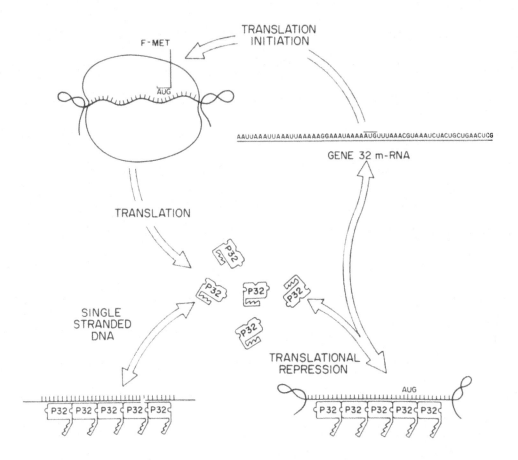

TRANSLATION
INITIATION

F-MET

AUG

AAUUAAAUUAAAUUAAAAAAGGAAAUAAAAAAUGUUUAAACGUAAAUCUACUGCUGAACUCG

GENE 32 m-RNA

TRANSLATION

P32

P32   P32   P32

SINGLE
STRANDED
DNA

P32

TRANSLATIONAL
REPRESSION

AUG

{P32}{P32}{P32}{P32}{P32}

{P32}{P32}{P32}{P32}{P32}

FIGURE 7.   Early in T4 infection gene 32 is transcribed, the 32 mRNA is translated and gp32 is produced. The protein binds all available ssDNA and in so doing promotes replication and recombination. When the intracellular pool of ssDNA is saturated, gp32 specifically binds to its own mRNA and blocks translation. The gp32 bound gene 32 mRNA is stable and can be derepressed if more ssDNA becomes available. Such a regulatory network precisely controls the amount of gp32 to a minimal level for protection of all available ssDNA.

Russel et al.[13] suggested that gp32 might specifically bind its own message by recognizing a uniquely long unstructured region around the ribosome binding site. The DNA sequence around the translational initiation region of gene 32 has recently been reported by Krisch et al.[76] and is shown above. This sequence is less structured than randomly generated sequences of equal length.[77] In fact, this region has no stable potential secondary structure.[77] The unstructured domain extends significantly beyond the AUG in the 3' direction. This finding is consistent with the hypothesis of coevolution[14] of the mRNA operator sequence and cooperative binding of gp32 which utilizes amino acid residues coded for by the unstructured sequence 3' to the AUG.

gp32 for single-stranded nucleic acids to explain the wide variety of in vivo and in vitro activities associated with this protein. The reactions of gp32 in vitro must reflect the role of gp32 in vivo for events that require the participation of a single-stranded nucleic acid binding protein. We envision the following events occurring in vivo. Early during T4 infection the free gp32 concentration is sufficient to bind cooperatively single-stranded DNA created either at replication forks or by repair-type events. This binding will facilitate strand displacement reactions at replication forks and protect all single-stranded DNA from nuclease digestion; these processes may also stimulate recombination between homologous DNA sequences. Once the level of single-stranded DNA reaches a maximum, the free concentration of gp32 will increase only until it reaches the concentration required for binding single-stranded RNA. Since the ribosome binding site of gene 32 mRNA may be uniquely single-stranded, compared to the other T4 sequences, gp32 will bind and saturate that domain of gene 32 mRNA, thus obstructing further translation. Although many experiments suggest that the known binding parameters of gp32 to single-stranded nucleic acids may be sufficient to explain all the in vivo functions of this protein (as above), some experiments do suggest that gp32 interacts with other proteins during T4 replication and recombination. We now consider the biochemical and genetic data for specific interactions of gp32 with a wide variety of other T4 (and *E. coli*) proteins.

A. DNA Polymerase

The central protein in the T4 replication complex is the T4 DNA polymerase, the product of gene 43. We have noted that gp32 stimulates DNA synthesis by the T4 DNA polymerase when assayed on a single-stranded DNA template.[19] Conversely, the *E. coli* and bacteriophage T7 single-stranded DNA binding proteins do not stimulate DNA synthesis by the T4 DNA polymerase. [58,60] As we have noted, the lack of stimulation by heterologous single-stranded DNA binding proteins might be a consequence of the different geometry of the complexes between the various binding proteins and DNA. More interestingly, one can imagine that the homologous reaction involves a protein-protein contact between gp43 and gp32. Such a complex has been isolated and studied.[19,59] Purified T4 DNA polymerase will co-migrate with gp32 multimers in a sucrose gradient at high gp32 concentrations. The formation of this complex is dependent on the presence of the T4 DNA polymerase; no associations are observed between gp32 and *E. coli* DNA polymerase I or II. This association of polymerase and gp32 has been shown to require an intact carboxyterminus of the gene 32 protein.[59]

B. RNA Primase

To obtain maximum DNA replication in vivo and in vitro, the products of genes 41 and 61 are required.[50,52,64,78] These genes code for proteins required to synthesize RNA oligomers that are used to prime DNA synthesis of the lagging strand of a replication fork.[50,64] Gene 32 protein may have an important role in this reaction by interacting directly with the gene 61 product. In vitro, the gene 61 protein has been shown to co-purify with the gene 32 protein.[59] Purified gp61 and gp32 also co-sediment as a complex in sucrose gradients and coelute during gel filtration chromatography. The complex between gp61 and gp32 is similar to that between gp32 and T4 DNA polymerase in that the carboxyterminus of gene 32 is required. In fact, when the carboxyterminus of gp32 is missing (to make P32*I), the altered gene 32 protein inhibits reactions stimulated by the primase proteins.[59,79] P32*I inhibits RNA primer synthesis by gp41 and gp61 on single-stranded DNA templates. RNA primer synthesis is not restored by the addition of the remaining accessory proteins. The authors suggest that the carboxyterminus of gp32 moderates the denaturation potential of gp32 such that primers are not displaced, i.e. melted off the template strand.

Mosig has studied the effects of gene 32 missense mutants on DNA synthesis that occurs in vivo, when the T4 RNA primase activity is eliminated by a mutation in gene 61.[22] This can be done because infections with amber mutations in gene 61, in an su⁻ host, manage to make substantial amounts of DNA in the absence of the primase polypeptide. Infections by phage that carry an amber mutation in gene 61, along with one of several missense mutations in gene 32, have been analyzed. One such double (*ts* L171/61⁻) gives no DNA synthesis (even though, under the conditions used, *ts* L171/61⁺ yields high level replication). Although one might consider the *ts* L171 site on gp32 to reside in a domain that interacts with gp61, we think the data are more consistent with the idea that *ts* L171 is in a portion of gp32 whose activity is especially crucial when *gp61 is missing* from the infected cell. Such metabolic dependencies, rather than "protein-protein interactions", are frequently a reasonable interpretation of genetic experiments.

The product of gene 41 is also required for the in vitro RNA priming of lagging-strand synthesis. Mosig et al.[21] have suggested that gp32 interacts with gp41. This is based on the preliminary finding that replication of parental DNA of 41⁻ mutants is differentially affected when various 41⁻/32^ts double mutants are examined. We note that the one gene 32 *ts* mutation which shows a unique response to gene 41 mutations is the above mentioned *ts* L171.

C. DNA Ligase
1. T4 DNA Ligase

Mosig has postulated that gp32 interacts with T4 DNA ligase.[80] This idea is based on two observations: (1) a missense mutation in gene 32 (*ts* L171) is weakly suppressed by mutations (including deletions) in the T4 genes rIIA and rIIB; and (2) the suppression effect is dependent on host DNA ligase. It is known that rII⁻ mutants suppress the lethality of mutations in T4 DNA ligase. That is, T4 lig⁻/rII⁻ mutants are viable while T4 lig⁻ is lethal.[81] Functional host DNA ligase is required for rII⁻ suppression of T4 lig⁻ mutants.[82] Mosig has argued that because rII mutations suppress *ts* L171, and because this suppression is also dependent on host ligase, gp32 interacts with T4 DNA ligase, and *ts* L171 is specifically defective in this interaction.[80]

However, this "suppression" is not very efficient. The double mutant *ts* L171/rII⁻ has not been demonstrated to be viable under any conditions that are restrictive for *ts* L171 alone. There is a small increase observed in the burst size (phage yield per infected bacterium) at the restrictive temperature (42°), and analysis of intracellular T4 DNA produced at 42°C indicated that the DNA of the *ts* L171/rII⁻ infection contained fewer single-stranded interruptions (gaps and/or nicks) than did intracellular DNA from a parallel infection of *ts* L171. This latter finding is consistent with increased ligase *activity* in the rII⁻ infection. The evidence for host ligase involvement in this phenomenon of weak suppression is not strong. Mosig and Breschkin[80] show that the burst size of *ts* L171/rII⁻ is lower at 42°C, on a host with a mutation in *E. coli* DNA ligase (lig⁻), than on a wild type (lig⁺) host. However, the lig⁺ and lig⁻ hosts compared are not isogenic. The lig⁺ host is *E. coli* strain B, while the lig⁻ strain, N2668, is a derivative of *E. coli* strain K12.[83] This strain difference is potentially significant in light of the involvement of the rII mutations, because rII mutants have different phenotypes on K and B strains.[84] Indeed, suppression of T4 ligase defects by mutations in rII shows strain specificity.[85] In order to demonstrate unambiguously involvement of host ligase in the *ts* L171/rII⁻ phenomenon, the comparison between lig⁺ and lig⁻ hosts ought to be made using *isogenic* strains.

Should the involvement of host ligase in the rII effect on *ts* L171 be adequately demonstrated, it would not require an explanation invoking direct protein-protein interactions between gp32 and T4 DNA ligase. We would suggest an alternative interpretation of such a result. The defect in *ts* L171 might result in an accumulation of single-stranded interruptions (gaps and/or nicks) on newly synthesized DNA, thus creating a greater demand for those enzymes (including ligase) which are involved in sealing such interruptions. *Indirect* metabolic enhancement of host ligase activity could somewhat ameliorate this defect. For example, rII⁻ infections could provide increased levels of dXTPs to the host DNA repair system (which must include *E. coli* DNA ligase). This would increase the activity of this host system. In light of such metabolic possibilities, we wish to point out that rII⁻ mutations also weakly suppress DNA synthesis defects resulting from mutations in two other T4 genes, x and y.[86]

2. E. coli DNA ligase

As noted above, T4 lig⁻/rII⁻ double mutants are viable on some hosts which have normal ligase activity. Karam et al.[87] selected T4 suppressor mutations which permitted a T4 lig⁻/rII⁻ mutant to grow on a host with a low level of ligase activity. Some of these suppressor mutants produced an altered gp32. The altered polypeptide displayed a slightly greater mobility in SDS polyacrylamide gels, consistent with a reduction in molecular weight of 1,000 daltons. It was suggested that this altered polypeptide might arise from nonsense, frameshift, or deletion mutations in the carboxyterminal end of gene 32. The alteration of the carboxyterminus of gp32 was proposed to alter an interaction between gp32 and host ligase and therefore result in increased host ligase activity, allowing growth of the T4 lig⁻/ rII⁻ mutant. However, no complementation analysis has been performed to show that the suppression is indeed brought about by the altered gene 32 product. In the absence of such a demonstration and without an understanding of the type of lesion which causes suppression, the conclusion that gp32 participates in an interaction with host ligase is somewhat premature. For example, none of these results eliminate the possibility that the target for suppressor isolation is near, but not in, gene 32. *Deletion* mutations knocking out this target gene might sometimes extend into gene 32 as well. Mutations which appear not to affect gene 32 (which are in the majority) might then be hits affecting only the target gene. Further characterization of these interesting mutations may distinguish between these possibilities.

In conclusion, we find, to date, no strong evidence for the notion that there are direct and specific protein-protein interactions between gp32 and either T4 or *E. coli* DNA ligase.

D. A T4-Encoded DNA Helicase

Snustad[88] suggested from genetic experiments that the gene 32 protein was unique among the proteins involved in DNA replication. Stoichiometric rather than catalytic amounts of protein were required for phage growth (also see Gold et al.[11]). The requirement for large quantities of protein may explain the lack of growth of gene 32 amber mutants on weak ochre suppressing strains.[89,90] Little[89] isolated mutations that permitted amber mutants in gene 32 to grow on ochre suppressing hosts. These second-site mutations, called sud (*sup*-*presses* *u*nwinding protein *d*eficiency), map in the gene 39 — gene 56 interval of T4. Interestingly, sud⁻ infections are delayed in the onset of rapid DNA replication.[89] Recent experimental evidence suggests that the *sud* gene may be identical to gene *dda*.[91] The *dda* gene product is a single-stranded DNA-dependent ATPase that has the ability to unwind double stranded DNA.[92,93] Enzymes that have this activity have been called "DNA helicases".[94] Perhaps the absence of this helicase activity in Sud⁻ infections reduces the rate of DNA synthesis by lowering the rate of helix unwinding, and thus ssDNA production; now the low level of gp32 present in amber mutant infections of ochre suppressing strains may be sufficient to protect available ssDNA and thus allow DNA synthesis to occur.

In this instance, there appears to be no reason to postulate protein-protein interactions between gp32 and the helicase. Although such an interaction is not ruled out, there is no evidence for its occurrence. A plausible model for sud⁻ suppression of gene 32 ambers on ochre suppressing strains can be based on known biochemical properties of gp32 and the sud-controlled helicase, without reference to protein-protein interactions.

E. Recombination Nucleases: T4 46/47 Nuclease and *E. coli* recBC Nuclease

Genes 46 and 47 of T4 code for, or control the activity of, a nuclease which is involved in T4 DNA recombination.[8,51,95-97] Mosig and Bock[98] have suggested that gp32 (specifically the carboxyterminus of the protein) interacts with this nuclease and "moderates" its degradative activity. A similar interaction with the recBC nuclease of *E. coli* is also postulated. Mosig and Bock[98] examined abortive infections of five mutants of gene 32 under restrictive conditions (at 42°C for *ts* mutants and on nonsuppressing host strains in the case of amber mutants). They observed that all mutants synthesized some DNA as measured by incorporation of ³H-thymidine into TCA precipitable material. In three mutant infections (*ts* G26, *am* A453, and *am* E315), a portion of this DNA was subsequently degraded. In two mutant infections (*ts* P7 and *ts* L171), degradation was not observed. Degradation of newly synthesized DNA was greatly reduced or eliminated when the infecting phage carried a second mutation in gene 46 and the infected host carried a mutation in the recB gene. In the same study, the fate of prelabeled ^{32}P *parental* DNA was examined in infections under those restrictive conditions. The results observed correlated well with the observations on the stability of newly synthesized DNA. Mutants *ts* P7 and *ts* L171 showed little degradation of parental DNA, while significant degradation was observed in infections with *ts* G26, *am* A453, and *am* E315. Again, this degradation was reduced or eliminated by mutational inactivation of the 46/47 nuclease and the recBC nuclease. The "degradation-insensitive" mutations *ts* P7 and *ts* L171 are more aminoterminal than *ts* G26. Additionally, the truncated polypeptides produced by the unsuppressed mutants *am* A453 and *am* E315 lack the carboxyterminal portion of the protein. It was therefore suggested that the wild type (intact) carboxyterminal portion of gp32 interacts with recBC nuclease and 46/47 nuclease and that this interaction protects DNA from degradation.[98]

These data are open to other interpretations. In this experiment, the total accumulation of progeny (newly replicated) DNA was measured over time. Labeled thymidine is continuously present. Degradation was defined as a decline over time in total incorporation from an early peak of total accumulation. Thus what is actually being measured is a result of relative rates of synthesis and degradation.

A more appropriate experiment would have been to pulse-label, chase, and follow the fate of incorporated radioactivity over time. This would allow a measurement of stability uniquely dependent on the rate of degradation. There is an additional difficulty with these experiments. The infections take place under restrictive conditions and, with the exception of *ts* L171, all of these mutant infections synthesize very small amounts of DNA. This DNA is tacitly assumed to be T4 DNA, but may not be. Cascino et al.[99] observed that, following infection of a restrictive host, a T4 double mutant (T$_4$ DNA polymerase$^-$/T$_4$ DNA ligase$^-$) synthesized a small but significant amount of DNA. This DNA was also subject to degradation, and degradation was blocked by a mutation in gene 46. Hybridization experiments showed that 96% of this DNA was homologous to *E. coli* DNA; *only 4% hybridized to T4 DNA.* Synthesis of this DNA was reported to occur in the absence of functional gp32.[99] It is thus possible that DNA labeled with thymidine in the Mosig and Bock experiments might contain a large fraction of host sequences.

The experimental problems cited above make it difficult to interpret the results on the synthesis and stability of *progeny* DNA. The nature of this DNA, its rate of synthesis, and rate of degradation are all unknown for each mutant infection. The conclusions based on these results should therefore be considered rather speculative. On the other hand, the experiments measuring degradation of prelabeled, *parental* DNA molecules are not subject to these difficulties. If one eliminates from consideration the data for progeny DNA, the data on stability of parental DNA give rise to at least one interpretation devoid of specific protein-protein interactions. We propose that the degradation of parental DNA is coupled to its replication. Specifically, in 32$^-$ infections an aberrant leading strand synthesis occurs, driven not by the gp32 stimulated stand displacement reaction of Figure 6 but driven directly by *degradation* of the displaced single-stranded DNA. This displaced strand is not copied and/or protected due to the lack of functional gp32. That DNA, the usual template for lagging strand synthesis, is thus degraded. This degradation might involve attack by the 46/47 nuclease and recBC nuclease.

It has been shown by Mosig and collaborators[41,98,100] that a significant fraction of parental DNA undergoes one round of replication in all 32 mutant infections with the exception of *ts* P7. Thus *ts* G26, *am* A453, and *am* E315 all replicate an appreciable fraction of parental template and a correspondingly high fraction of the parental DNA is degraded. The mutant *ts* P7 shows little replication of parental DNA and that parental chromosome remains largely undegraded. Our model is inconsistent (at first glance) with the results from only one mutant, *ts* L171 (and wild type). The mutant *ts* L171 and wild type both replicate significant portions of parental DNA and yet show little degradation of that parental template. In the case of wild type, one doesn't find this to be surprising. In the case of *ts* L171, it is surprising, at least initially. However, Mosig and Breschkin[41] have shown that in contrast to all other conditional lethal mutations in gene 32, *ts* L171 shows significant accumulation of stable DNA at restrictive conditions. In fact, at 42° *ts* L171 synthesizes about 20% the amount of DNA made by wild type in a parallel infection. It is also the least restrictive of the classical gene 32 *ts* mutations.[40] It is probable that the growth defect in *ts* L171 at 42° is not due to an absolute DNA replication block, as suggested by Mosig and Breschkin.[80] We propose that at 42°C *ts* L171 does synthesize the lagging (as well as leading) strand to a significant extent. Thus, under our model, degradation of parental DNA (which results from failure to copy or protect the displaced strand) would not be observed. In this sense, we are proposing that *ts* L171 is fundamentally different than the other classical *ts* alleles of gene 32. We will return to this notion in the final portion of this section. For now, we point out that much of the genetic underpinnings for postulated protein-protein interactions involving gp32 can be considered to be anomolies in the behavior of *ts* L171 by itself or in combination with gene 61, gene 41 (B above), rII (C above) and now 46/47 mutants.

In conclusion, we suggest that these data do support the in vivo and in vitro findings that gp32 bound DNA is protected against digestion by a variety of nucleases, including recBC and 46/47 nuclease, but no specific protein-protein contacts between gp32 and this array of nucleases are required to envision protection mechanisms.

F. Others

Mosig and collaborators[20-22,101] have postulated an ultra-glamorous model of gp32 function, including interactions between gp32 and the products of genes 39 and 52 (components of the T4 DNA gyrase), gene 17 (involved in DNA packaging), and genes rIIA and rIIB. This model suggests that nearly all replication and recombination proteins interact with the gene 32 protein in specific ways and that temperature sensitive and amber mutations in gene 32 are altered in particular interactions. It is not the purpose of this article to review all the aspects of the Mosig model. For the present, we consider these interesting ideas to be speculative in nature, awaiting further experimental results that may confirm or refute what appear in many cases to be preliminary observations. For those readers interested in the details of this model, we note Mosig et al.[20,22]

G. Summary and Caveat

After critical examination of the literature on protein-protein interactions involving gp32, we must conclude that there is no firm experimental evidence for a wide array of protein contacts involving gp32. However, gp32 might interact directly with T4 DNA polymerase and at least one component of T4 RNA primase (gp61). We will consider below (Part V) some implications of these specific contacts.

In considering the genetic data regarding protein-protein interactions, we have been impressed by two things. One is the recurring possibility that results suggestive of protein-protein interactions often lend themselves to plausible alternative interpretations based on indirect, metabolic connections. The second is the near ubiquity of the gene 32 missense mutation *ts* L171 in genetic arguments supporting specific protein-protein interactions. As stated above, it is possible that *ts* L171 is fundamentally different from the other classical *ts* alleles of gene 32. We have already pointed out some obvious differences. We now wish to mention another unique property of this mutant. The mutant strain of *E. coli* Tab324[42] is unusually restrictive for missense mutations in gene 32. While *ts* L171 is the *least* restrictive of the classical missense mutations in gene 32 when assayed on *E. coli* B (and the Tab+ parent of Tab324) it is the *most* restrictive mutation when growth is assayed on Tab 324 (Table 2). The difference is quite dramatic. While *ts* L171 grows well on Tab+ even at

Table 2
PLATING EFFICIENCIES OF THE CLASSICAL GENE 32
MISSENSE MUTATIONS ON Tab324 AND NapIV

	25°C		37°C		42°C	
	NapIV[a]	Tab324	NapIV	Tab324	NapIV	Tab324
ts P7	1.00^{b}	0.50	$<10^{-2}$	$<10^{-4}$	$<10^{-4}$	$<10^{-4}$
ts L171	1.00	$<10^{-4}$	0.95	$<10^{-4}$	$<10^{-4}$	$<10^{-4}$
ts G26	1.00	0.73	0.31	$<10^{-4}$	$<10^{-4}$	$<10^{-4}$
ts P401	1.00	0.82	$<10^{-2}$	$<10^{-4}$	$<10^{-4}$	$<10^{-4}$

[a] NapIV (Tab^{+}) is the parental strain of the Tab324 mutant.
[b] Efficiency of plaque formation with the NapIV at 25°C value defined as 1.

37°C, it is lethal on Tab^{-} at 25°C and all higher temperatures. At low temperature on Tab^{-}, ts L171 directs DNA synthesis at a high rate, yet no plaque is formed.[41] This DNA must be unacceptable as a phage genome. This mutant is different from the other classical mutations which show a more straightforward relationship between the level of DNA synthesis and the progeny yield. We do not yet know, at a biochemical level, the defect in the ts L171 protein; we might suggest that its peculiar biochemistry leads to substantial, but aberrant, lagging strand synthesis. In any case, we are wary of putative protein-protein interactions postulated solely on the basis of the peculiarities of this one missense mutation.

V. FUNCTION OF gp32 AT A REPLICATION FORK

We have summarized the in vivo and in vitro experiments that establish the importance of the gene 32 protein in T4 DNA replication. Here we extract from this information a model for the actions of gp32. Our model, which is quite simple and unglamorous, emphasizes those functions of gp32 that are probably shared by other single-stranded DNA binding proteins and offers some suggestions for future research into this class of proteins.

The most important functions of gp32 are facilitation of strand displacement, stimulation of lagging strand synthesis, and protection of ssDNA against nucleolytic attack. Facilitation of strand displacement must depend (minimally) on the capacity of gp32 to fill quickly (as in Figure 6) a short single-stranded segment of DNA, presumably by utilization of the large cooperativity displayed by gp32. Additional contributions might be made if gp32 interacts meaningfully with DNA polymerase. We note that only a particular model for leading strand synthesis, in which gp43 binds gp32 so as to alter the carboxyterminus (equivalent to removal of the A peptide), utilized gp32 to "unwind" double helical DNA.[30,59] The suggestion is plausible but we are not drawn to the formulation. DNA polymerase, as well as the replication accessory proteins, the T4 DNA helicase,[92,93] and the T4 topoisomerase,[102,103] each contribute to DNA unwinding; if gp32 ever directly opens a replication fork, that act is aided by components that can partially denature the DNA and eliminate the kinetic block against denaturation by gp32. In fact, the facilitation of strand displacement that we presently perceive does not depend on gp32 participation in a multiple peptide, oligomeric complex (Figure 6).

Facilitation of lagging strand synthesis must depend (minimally) on the capacity of gp32 to hold the bases of the template in an appropriate configuration for DNA polymerase action; further contributions are certainly made by the capacity of gp32 to denature weak hairpins in the lagging strand template.[66,67] Additionally, if gp32 interacts meaningfully with the T4 primase (gp61), further contributions might be made toward the rate of primer synthesis and use. With or without a direct interaction with gp61, the displaced strand is probably always covered by binding protein; the intrinsic binding constant, the cooperativity, and the intracellular concentration of free gp32 guarantee that saturation. The complex between gp32 and the displaced strand may serve as either a template for lagging strand synthesis or an invasive element for recombination.[104] Whatever the fate of the displaced strand, gp32 certainly protects that DNA against nuclease attack.

The gene 32 protein has not been shown to contain domains as traditionally defined, although the carboxyterminus may be found to possess an independent activity. However, many partial reactions of gp32 are worthy of detailed study, especially if the structure of gp32 is ultimately solved. One would like to know the relationship between the elements that participate in DNA contacts and those that participate in the protein-protein interactions that provide cooperativity. The evolution of cooperativity may well have occurred as translational regulation developed; does cooperativity utilize elements of gp32 other than the very aminoterminus? Are there differences in protein conformation when gp32 resides on either a short oligonucleotide or a long polynucleotide? What is the basis for discrimination against RNA relative to DNA (since binding to RNA plays a regulatory role)? Along these lines, one would love to understand the biological role of the autogenous translational regulation; the suggestions offered thus far are not satisfactory.[14] Lastly, if gp32 interacts directly with either DNA polymerase or a primase subunit, the relationship between that binding and the conformation of the carboxyterminlus (the A peptide) should be fascinating. The gene 32 protein has a variety of interesting activities, and we look forward to further research on it and other DNA-binding proteins.

ACKNOWLEDGMENTS

We thank Mary Anne Nelson, Britta S. Singer, Gary Stormo, Peter von Hippel, and Ken Williams for helpful discussions and information received prior to publication. This work was supported by the NIH (GM#19963).

REFERENCES

1. **Wood, W. B. and Revel, H. R.**, The genome of bacteriophage T4, *Bacteriol. Rev.*, 40, 847, 1976.
2. **Broker, T. R. and Doermann, A. H.**, Molecular and genetic recombination of bacteriophage T4, *Annu. Rev. Genet.*, 9, 213, 1976.
3. **Epstein, R. H., Bolle, A., Steinberg, C. M., Kellenberger, E., Boy de la Tour, E., Chevalley, R., Edgar, R. S., Sussman, M., Denhardt, G. H., and Lielausis, I.**, Physiological studies of conditional lethal mutants of bacteriophage T4D, *Cold Spring Harbor Symp. Quant. Biol.*, 28, 375, 1963.
4. **Riva, S., Cascino, A., and Geiduschek, E. P.**, Coupling of late transcription to viral replication in bacteriophage T4, *J. Mol. Biol.*, 54, 85, 1970.
5. **Tomizawa, J.-I.**, Molecular mechanisms of genetic recombination in bacteriophage: joint molecules and their conversion to recombinant molecules, *J. Cell. Physiol.*, 70 (Suppl. 1), 201, 1967.
6. **Broker, T. R. and Lehman, I. R.**, Branched DNA molecules: intermediates in T4 recombination, *J. Mol. Biol.*, 60, 131, 1971.
7. **Kozinski, A. W. and Felgenhauer, Z. Z.**, Molecular recombination in T4 bacteriophage deoxyribonucleic acid. II. Single strand breaks and exposure of uncomplemented areas as a prerequisite for recombination, *J. Virol.*, 1, 1193, 1967.
8. **Berger, H., Warren, A. J., and Fry, K. E.**, Variations in genetic recombination due to amber mutations in T4D bacteriophage, *J. Virol.*, 3, 171, 1969.
9. **Baldy, M. W.**, The UV-sensitivity of some early function temperature-sensitive mutants of phage T4, *Virology*, 40, 272, 1970.

10. **Wu, J-R. and Yeh, Y-C.,** Requirement of a functional gene 32 product of bacteriophage T4 in UV repair, *J. Virol.,* 12, 758, 1973.

11. **Gold L., O'Farrell, P. Z., and Russell, M.,** Regulation of gene 32 expression during bacteriophage T4 infection of *Escherichia coli, J. Biol. Chem.,* 251, 7251, 1976.

12. **Krisch, H., Bolle, A., and Epstein, R. H.,** Regulation of the synthesis of bacteriophage T4 gene 32 protein, *J. Mol. Biol.,* 88, 89, 1974.

13. **Russel, M. L., Gold, L., Morrissett, H., and O'Farrell, P. Z.,** Translational autogenous regulation of gene 32 during bacteriophage T4 infection, *J. Biol. Chem.,* 251, 7263, 1976.

14. **Lemaire, G., Gold, L., and Yarus, M.,** Autogenous translational repression of bacteriophage T4 gene 32 expression *in vitro, J. Mol. Biol.,* 126, 73, 1978.

15. **Alberts, B. and Frey, L.,** T4 bacteriophage gene 32: a structural protein in the replication and recombination of DNA, *Nature,* 227, 1313, 1970.

16. **Kowalczykowski, S. C., Lonberg, N., Newport, J. W., and von Hippel, P. H.,** Interactions of bacteriophage T4-coded gene 32 protein with nucleic acids. I. Characterization of the binding interactions, *J. Mol. Biol.,* 145, 75, 1981.

17. **Newport, J., Lonberg, N., Kowalczykowski, S. C., and von Hippel, P.,** Interactions of T4-coded gene 32 protein with nucleic acids. II. Specificity of binding to DNA and RNA, *J. Mol. Biol.,* 145, 105, 1981.

18. **Alberts, B. M.,** DNA-unwinding proteins and their role in the replication of DNA, in *Mechanism and Regulation of DNA Replication,* Kolber, A. R. and Kohiyama, M., Eds., Plenum Press, New York, 1974, 133.

19. **Huberman, J., Kornberg, A., and Alberts, B.,** Stimulation of T4 bacteriophage DNA polymerase by the protein product of T4 gene 32, *J. Mol. Biol.,* 62, 39, 1971.

20. **Mosig, G., Dannenberg, R., Ghosal, D., Luder, A., Benedict, S., and Bock, S.,** General genetic recombination in bacteriophage T4, in *Stadler Symp.,* Vol. 3, Redei, G., Ed., University of Missouri, Columbia, 1979, 31.

21. **Mosig, G., Dannenberg, R., Benedict, S., Luder, A., and Bock, S.,** T4 DNA replication, in Microbiology 1980, Schlessinger, D., Ed., *Society for Microbiology,* Washington, D.C., 1980, 254.

22. **Mosig, G., Luder, A., Garcia, G., Dannenberg, R., and Bock, S.,** *In vivo* interactions of genes and proteins in DNA replication and recombination of phage T4, *Cold Spring Harbor Symp. Quant. Biol.,* 43, 501, 1978.

23. **Kowalczykowski, S. C., Bear, D. G., and von Hippel, P. H.,** Single-stranded DNA binding proteins, in *The Enzymes,* Vol. 14a, Boyer, P., Ed., Academic Press, New York, 1981, chap. 21.

24. **Williams, K. R. and Konigsberg, W.,** DNA helix-destabilizing proteins, in *Gene Amplification and Analysis,* Vol. II, Chirikjian, J. and Pappas, T., Eds., Elsevier Press, Amsterdam, 1981, 476.

25. **Alberts, B., Amodio, F. J., Jenkins, M., Gutman, E. D., and Ferris, F. L.,** Studies with DNA cellulose chromatography. I. DNA-binding proteins from *Escherichia coli, Cold Spring Harbor Symp. Quant. Biol.,* 33, 289, 1968.

26. **Delius, H., Mantell, N. J., and Alberts, B.,** Characterization by electron microscopy of the complex formed between T4 bacteriophage gene 32-protein and DNA, *J. Mol. Biol.,* 67, 341, 1972.

27. **Kirschner, K. and Bisswanger, H.,** Multifunctional proteins, *Annu. Rev. Biochem.,* 45, 143, 1976.

28. **Pabo, C. O., Sauer, R. T., Sturtevant, J. M., and Ptashne, M.,** The lambda repressor contains two domains, *Proc. Natl. Acad. Sci. U.S.A.,* 76, 1608, 1979.

29. **Sauer, R. T., Pabo, C. O., Meyer, B. J., Ptashne, M., and Backman, K. C.,** Regulatory functions of the λ repressor reside in amino-terminal domain, *Nature,* 279, 396, 1979.

30. **Moise, H. and Hosoda, J.,** T4 gene 32 protein model for control of activity at replication fork, *Nature,* 259, 455, 1976.

31. **Williams, K. R. and Konigsberg, W. H.,** Structural changes in the T4 gene 32 protein induced by DNA and polynucleotides, *J. Biol. Chem.,* 253, 2463, 1978.

32. **Hosoda, J. and Moise, H.,** Purification and physico-chemical properties of limited proteolysis products of T4 helix destabilizing protein (gene 32 protein), *J. Biol. Chem.,* 253, 7547, 1978.

33. **Spicer, E. K., Williams, K. R., and Konigsberg, W. H.,** T4 gene 32 protein trypsin-generated fragments: fluorescence measurements of DNA-binding parameters, *J. Biol. Chem.,* 254, 6433, 1979.

34. **Lonberg, N., Kowalczykowski, S. C., Paul, L. S., and von Hippel, P. H.,** Interactions of bacteriophage T4 encoded gene 32 protein with nucleic acids. III. Binding properties of two specific proteolytic digestion products of the protein (G32P*I and G32P*III), *J. Mol. Biol.,* 145, 123, 1981.

35. **Hosoda, J., Takacs, B., and Brack, C.,** Denaturation of T4 DNA by an *in vitro* processed gene 32 protein, *FEBS Lett.,* 47, 338, 1977. 1974.

36. **Jensen, D. E., Kelly, R. C., and von Hippel, P.,** DNA "melting" proteins II. Effects of bacteriophage T4 gene 32 protein binding on the conformation and stability of nucleic acid structures, *J. Biol. Chem.,* 251, 7215, 1976.

37. **Williams, K., LoPresti, M., and Setoguchi, M.,** Primary structure of the bacteriophage T4 helix-destabilizing protein, *J. Biol. Chem.,* 256, 1754, 1981.

38. **Sancar, A., Williams, K. R., Chase, J. W., and Rupp, W. D.,** Sequences of the *ssb* gene and protein, *Proc. Natl. Acad. Sci. U.S.A.,* 78, 4274, 1981.

39. **Dunn, J. J. and Studier, F. W.,** Nucleotide sequence from the genetic left end of bacteriophage T7 DNA to the beginning of gene 4, *J. Mol. Biol.,* 148, 303, 1981.

40. **Mosig, G., Berquist, W., and Bock, S.,** Multiple interactions of a DNA binding protein *in vivo.* III. Phage T4 gene 32 mutations differentially affect insertion-type recombination and membrane properties, *Genetics,* 86, 5, 1977.

41. **Breschkin, A. M. and Mosig, G.,** Multiple interactions of a DNA-binding protein in vivo. I. Gene 32 mutations of phage T4 inactivate different steps in DNA replication and recombination, *J. Mol. Biol.,* 112, 279, 1977.

42. **Nelson, M. A.,** personal communication, 1981.

43. **McPherson, A., Jurnak, F. A., Wang, A. H. J., Molineux, I., and Rich, A.,** Structure at 2.3A resolution of the gene 5 product of bacteriophage fd: a DNA unwinding protein, *J. Mol. Biol.,* 134, 379, 1979.

44. **Coleman, J. E. and Oakley, J. L.,** Physical chemical studies of the structure and function of DNA binding (helix destabilizing) proteins, *Crit. Rev. Biochem.,* 7, 247, 1979.

45. **Coleman, J. E., Anderson, R. A., Ratcliffe, R. G., and Armitage, I. M.,** Structure of gene 5 protein-oligodeoxynucleotide complexes as determined by ^{1}H, ^{19}F, and ^{31}P nuclear magnetic resonance, *Biochemistry,* 15, 5419, 1976.

46. **Anderson, R. A. and Coleman, J. E.,** Physicochemical properties of DNA binding proteins: gene 32 protein of T4 and *Escherichia coli* unwinding protein, *Biochemistry,* 14, 5485, 1975.

47. **Curtiss, M. J. and Alberts, B.,** Studies on the structure of intracellular bacteriophage T4 DNA, *J. Mol. Biol.,* 102, 793, 1976.

48. **Mufti, S.,** The effect on ultraviolet mutagenesis of genes 32, 41, 44, and 45 alleles of phage T4 in the presence of wild-type or antimutator DNA polymerase, *Virology,* 105, 345, 1980.

49. **Watanabe, S. and Goodman, M. F.,** Mutator and antimutator phenotypes of suppressed amber mutants in genes 32, 41, 44, 45 and 62 in bacteriophage T4, *J. Virol.,* 25, 73, 1978.

50. **Liu, C. C., Burke, R. L., Hibner, U., Barry, J., and Alberts, B. M.,** Probing DNA replication with the T4 bacteriophage *in vitro* system, *Cold Spring Harbor Symp. Quant. Biol.,* 43, 469, 1978.

51. **Broker, T. R.,** An electron microscopic analysis of pathways for bacteriophage T4 DNA recombination, *J. Mol. Biol.,* 81, 1, 1973.

52. **Nossal, N. G. and Peterlin, B. M.,** DNA replication by bacteriophage T4 proteins, *J. Biol. Chem.,* 254, 6032, 1979.

53. **Greve, J., Maestre, M. F., Mise, H., and Hosoda, J.,** Circular dichroism study of the interaction between T4 gene 32 protein and polyneuclotides, *Biochemistry,* 17, 887, 1978.

54. **Huang, W. M. and Lehman, I. R.,** On the exonuclease activity of phage T4 deoxyribonucleic acid polymerase, *J. Biol. Chem.,* 247, 3139, 1972.

55. **Gold, L., Lemaire, G., Martin, C., Morrissett, H., O'Conner, P., O'Farrell, P. Z., Russel, M., and Shapiro, R.,** Molecular aspects of gene 32 expression in *Escherichia coli* infected with the bacteriophage T4, in *Nucleic Acid-Protein Recognition,* Vogel, H. J., Ed., Academic Press, New York, 1977, 91.

56. **Taylor, A. and Smith, G. R.,** Unwinding and rewinding of DNA by the *recBC* enzyme, *Cell,* 22, 447, 1980.

57. **Sinha, N. K., Morris, C. F., and Alberts, B. M.,** Efficient *in vitro* replication of double-stranded DNA templates by a purified T4 bacteriophage replication system, *J. Biol. Chem.,* 255, 4290, 1980.

58. **Sigal, N., Delius, H., Kornberg, T., Gefter, M. L. and Alberts, B. M.,** A DNA unwinding protein isolated from Escherichia coli: its interaction with DNA and DNA polymerase, *Proc. Natl. Acad. Sci. U.S.A.,* 69, 3537, 1972.

59. **Burke, R. L., Alberts, B. M., and Alberts, B. M., and Hosoda, J.,** Proteolytic removal of the COOH terminus of the T4 gene 32 helix-destabilizing protein alters the T4 *in vitro* replication complex, *J. Biol. Chem.,* 255, 11484, 1980.

60. **Reuben, R. and Gefter, M. L.,** A deoxyribonucleic acid-binding protein induced by bacteriophage T7, *J. Biol. Chem.,* 249, 3843, 1974.

61. **Olivera, B. M., Scheffler, I. E., and Lehman, I. R.,** Enzymatic joining of polynucleotides. IV. Formation of a circular deoxyadenylate-deoxythymidylate copolymer, *J. Mol. Biol.,* 36, 275, 1968.

62. **Gillin, F. D. and Nossal, N.,** Control of mutation frequency by bacteriophage T4 DNA polymerase. I. The CB120 antimutator DNA polymerase is defective in strand displacement, *J. Biol. Chem.,* 251, 5219, 1976.

63. **Alberts, B., Barry, J., Bittner, M., Davies, M., Hamainaba, H., Liu, C. C., Mace, C., Moran, L., Morris, C. F., Piperno, J., and Sinha, N.,** *In vitro* DNA replication catalyzed by six purified T4 bacteriophage proteins, in *Nucleic Acid-Protein Recognition,* Vogel, H. J., Ed., Academic Press, New York, 1977, 31.

64. **Silver, L. L. and Nossal, N. G.,** DNA replication by bacteriophage T4 proteins: role of the DNA delay gene 61 in the chain-initiation reaction, *Cold Spring Harbor Symp. Quan. Biol.,* 43, 489, 1978.

65. **Newport, J. W., Kowalcyzkowski, S. C., Lonberg, N., Paul, L. S., and von Hippel, P.,** Molecular aspects of the interactions of T4 coded gene 32-protein and DNA polymerase (gene 43 protein) with nucleic acids, in *Mechanistic Studies of DNA Replication and Genetic Recombination: ICN-UCLA Symposia on Molecular and Cellular Biology,* Vol. 19, Alberts, B. M., Ed., Academic Press, New York, 1980, 449.

66. **Roth, A. C., Englund, P. T., and Nossal, N. G.,** DNA-dependent dNMP formation in a T4 replication complex: correlation with pauses in DNA synthesis, *Fed. Proc.,* 40, 1903, 1981.

67. **Huang, C. C., Hearst, J. E., and Alberts, B. M.,** Two types of replication proteins increase the rate at which T4 DNA polymerase traverses the helical regions in single-stranded DNA template, *J. Biol. Chem.,* 256, 4087, 1981.

68. **Nossal, N. G.,** DNA synthesis on a double-stranded DNA template by T4 bacteriophage DNA polymerase and the T4 gene 32 DNA unwinding protein, *J. Biol. Chem.,* 249, 5668, 1974.

69. **MacKay, V. and Linn, S.,** Selective inhibition of the DNase activity of the *recBC* enzyme by the DNA binding protein from *Escherichia coli, J. Biol. Chem.,* 251, 3716, 1976.

70. **O'Farrell, P. Z., Huang, W. M., and Gold, L. M.,** Identification of prereplicative bacteriophage T4 proteins, *J. Biol. Chem.,* 248, 5499, 1973.

71. **Vanderslice, R. W. and Yegian, C. D.,** The identification of late bacteriophage T4 proteins on sodium dodecyl sulfate polyacrylamide gels, *Virology,* 60, 265, 1974.

72. **O'Farrell, P. Z. and Gold, L. M.,** Bacteriophage T4 gene expression: evidence for two classes of prereplicative cistrons, *J. Biol. Chem.,* 248, 5502, 1973.

73. **Rabussay, D. and Geiduschek, E. P.,** Regulation of gene action in the development of lytic bacteriophages, in *Comprehensive Virology,* Vol. 8, Frankel-Conrat, H. and Wagner, R. R., Eds., Plenum Press, New York, 1977, chap. 1.

74. **Goldberger, R. F.,** Autogenous regulation of gene expression, *Science,* 183, 810, 1974.

75. **Gold, L., Pribnow, D., Schneider, T., Shinedling, S., Singer, B. S., and Stormo, G.,** Translational initiation in procaryotes, *Annu. Rev. Microbiol.,* 35, 365, 1981.

76. **Krisch, H. M., Duvoisin, R. M., Allet, B., and Epstein, R. H.,** A chimeric plasmid containing gene 32 of bacteriophage T4, in *Mechanistic Studies of DNA Replication and Recombination,* Alberts, B., Ed., Academic Press, New York, 1980, 501.

77. **von Hippel, P. H., Kowalczykowski, S. C., Lonberg, N., Newport, J. W., Paul, L. S., Stormo, G., and Gold, L.,** On the specificity of nucleic acid-protein interactions: the T4-coded gene 32 protein auto-regulatory system, in preparation, 1983.

78. **Yegian, C. D., Mueller, M., Selzer, G., Russo, V., and Stahl, F. W.,** Properties of DNA-delay mutants of bacteriophage T4, *Virology,* 46, 900, 1971.

79. **Hosoda, J., Burke, R. L., Moise, H., Kubota, I., and Tsugita, A.,** The control of T4 gene 32 helix-destabilizing protein activity in a DNA replication complex, in *Mechanistic Studies of DNA Replication and Genetic Recombination: ICN-UCLA Symposia on Molecular and Cellular Biology,* Alberts, B. M., Ed., Vol. 19, Academic Press, New York, 1980, 505.

80. **Mosig, G. and Breschkin, A. M.,** Genetic evidence for an additional function of T4 gene 32 protein: interaction with ligase, *Proc. Natl. Acad. Sci. U.S.A.,* 72, 1226, 1975.

81. **Berger, H. and Kozinski, A. W.,** Suppression of T4D ligase mutations by rIIA and rIIB mutations, *Proc. Natl. Acad. Sci. U.S.A.,* 64, 897, 1969.

82. **Gellert, M. and Bullock, M. L.,** DNA ligase mutants of *Escherichia coli, Proc. Natl. Acad. Sci. U.S.A.,* 67, 1580, 1970.

83. **Gottesman, M. M., Hicks, M. L., and Gellert, M.,** Genetics and function of DNA ligase in *Escherichia coli, J. Mol. Biol.,* 77, 531, 1973.

84. **Benzer, S.,** Fine structure of a genetic region in bacteriophage, *Proc. Natl. Acad. Sci. U.S.A.,* 41, 344, 1955.

85. **Karam, J. D. and Barker, B.,** Properties of bacteriophage T4 mutants defective in gene 30 (deoxyribonucleic acid ligase) and the rII gene, *J. Virol.,* 7, 260, 1971.

86. **Cunningham, R. P. and Berger, H.,** Mutations affecting genetic recombination in bacteriophage T4D. I. Pathway analysis, *Virology,* 80, 67, 1977.

87. **Karam, J. D., Leach, M., and Heere, L. J.,** Functional interactions between the DNA ligase of *Escherichia coli* and components of the DNA metabolic apparatus of T4 bacteriophage, *Genetics,* 91, 177, 1979.

88. **Snustad, D. P.,** Dominance interactions in *Escherichia coli* cells mixedly infected with bacteriophage T4D wild type and *amber* mutants and their possible implications as to type of gene-product function: catalytic vs. stoichiometric, *Virology,* 35, 550, 1968.

89. **Little, J.,** Mutants of bacteriophage T4 which allow amber mutants of gene 32 to grow in ochre-suppressing hosts, *Virology,* 53, 47, 1973.

90. **Floor, E.,** Interaction of morphogenetic genes of bacteriophage T4, *J. Mol. Biol.,* 47, 293, 1970.

91. **Gauss, P.,** unpublished data, 1981.

92. **Behme, M. T. and Ebisuzaki, K.,** Characterization of a bacteriophage T4 mutant lacking DNA-dependent ATPase, *J. Virol.,* 15, 50, 1975.

93. **Kuhn, B., Abdel-Monem, M., and Hoffmann-Berling, H.,** DNA helicases, *Cold Spring Harbor Symp. Quant. Biol.,* 43, 63, 1978.

94. **Geider, K. and Hoffmann-Berling, H.,** Proteins controlling the helical structure of DNA, *Annu. Rev. Biochem.,* 50, 233, 1981.

95. **Hosoda, J., Mathews, E., and Jansen, B.,** Role of genes 46 and 47 in bacteriophage T4 reproduction. I. *In vivo* deoxyribonucleic acid replication, *J. Virol.,* 8, 372, 1971.

96. **Kutter, E. M. and Wiberg, J. S.,** Degradation of cytosine-containing bacterial and bacteriophage DNA after infection of *Escherichia coli B* with bacteriophage T4D wild type and with mutants defective in genes 46, 47 and 56, *J. Mol. Biol.,* 38, 395, 1968.

97. **Mickelson, C. M. and Wiberg, J. S.,** Membrane-associated DNase activity controlled by genes 46 and 47 of bacteriophage T4D and elevated DNase activity associated with the T4 das mutation, *J. Virol.,* 40, 65, 1981.

98. **Mosig, G. and Bock, S.,** Gene 32 protein of bacteriophage T4 moderates the activities of the T4 gene 46/47 controlled nuclease and of the *Escherichia coli recBC* nuclease *in vivo, J. Virol.,* 17, 756, 1976.

99. **Cascino, A., Riva, S., and Geiduschek, E. P.,** Host DNA synthesis after infection of *Escherichia coli* with mutants of bacteriophage T4, *Virology,* 40, 403, 1971.

100. **Breschkin, A. M. and Mosig, G.,** Multiple interactions of a DNA-binding protein *in vivo.* II. Effects of host mutations on DNA replication of phage T4 and 32 mutants, *J. Mol. Biol.,* 112, 295, 1977.

101. **Mosig, G., Benedict, S., Ghosal, D., Luder, A., Dannenberg, R., and Bock, S.,** Genetic analysis of DNA replication in bacteriophage T4, in *Mechanistic Studies of DNA Replication and Recombination,* Alberts, B., Ed., Academic Press, New York, 1980, 527.

102. **Liu, L. F., Liu, C. C., and Alberts, B. M.,** T4 DNA topoisomerase: a new ATP dependent enzyme essential for initiation of T4 bacteriophage DNA replication, *Nature (London),* 281, 456, 1979.

103. **Stetler, G. L., King, G. L., and Huang, W. M.,** T4 DNA-delay proteins required for specific DNA replication, form a complex that has ATP-dependent DNA topoisomerase activity, *Proc. Natl. Acad. Sci. U.S.A.,* 76, 3737, 1979.

104. **Meselson, M. S. and Radding, C. M.,** A general model for genetic recombination, *Proc. Natl. Acad. Sci. U.S.A.,* 72, 358, 1975.

Chapter 5

REGULATION OF SYNTHESIS OF THE β & β' SUBUNITS OF RNA POLYMERASE OF *ESCHERICHIA COLI*

Rudolph Spangler and Geoffrey Zubay

TABLE OF CONTENTS

I. INTRODUCTION

Bacterial cells contain at least 1,000 copies of RNA polymerase. This single multiprotein complex is responsible for most of the transcription in *Escherichia coli*. It is also used in an unmodified or modified form for transcription of a large number of bacteriophage genes. The polymerase recognizes about a thousand different promoters on the bacterial chromosome with different efficiencies that depend upon the sequences of these promoters as well as more or less specific regulatory factors whose concentrations vary with the physiological state of the cell. This differential response in certain cases also extends to the sites of provisional terminators (attenuators) found in host and viral genes which are modulated by a variety of antiterminator factors. The complexity of the bacterial polymerase shown by its response to a wide variety of situations stretches the imagination to the very limits of biochemical reality. Superimposed on this functional complexity is the growing realization that the synthesis of the RNA polymerase itself is one of the more intricately regulated gene expression processes in *E. coli*. At the present time the regulatory processes which control RNA polymerase synthesis are only partly understood. As will be argued below, the regulatory mechanism which controls the amount of RNA polymerase reflects the desirability for RNA polymerase levels to be coupled with the cell's needs for ribosomal proteins.[1] The primary object of this paper is to describe the regulatory mechanism which controls the synthesis of the β and β′ subunits of RNA polymerase.

II. DESCRIPTION OF THE RNA POLYMERASE ENZYME

The central dogma, which states that DNA "makes" RNA and RNA "makes" protein, signaled biochemists to search for an RNA polymerizing activity. The first such enzyme, discovered by Ochoa and Grunberg-Manago, became known as polynucleotide phosphorylase. This enzyme linked ribonucleotide diphosphates into a polynucleotide chain with the correct 3′ to 5′ linkages found in naturally occurring RNA. It failed to show a requirement for a DNA template and, therefore, did not appear to be the key enzyme that was hypothesized to function in the DNA to protein pathway. The search continued and the finding of a DNA-requiring enzyme in liver extracts was soon followed by the discovery of comparable enzyme activities in bacterial extracts. This enzyme required a DNA template, Mg^{2+} or Mn^{2+}, and ribonucleotide triphosphate substrates. Hybridization studies showed that the RNA synthesized was complementary in composition to the DNA, thereby satisfying the demand made by the central dogma. Final proof that the enzyme was required for the in vivo synthesis of all major species of bacterial RNA came when it was shown that the highly specific antibiotic, rifamycin, and its synthetic analogue rifampicin, immediately stopped initiation of RNA synthesis, and that this effect was reversed in a mutant containing an altered RNA polymerase insensitive to the drug.

Early attempts to purify the enzyme led to the isolation of a tetramer containing two α subunits, one β subunit, and one β′ subunit with molecular weights of 44,000, 150,000, and 165,000 daltons, respectively. This enzyme was highly active in vitro when assayed with nicked template and a mixture of Mg^{2+} and Mn^{2+} divalent cations. Enzyme activity was greatly reduced when nicked template was replaced by intact DNA. High activity could be restored in the presence of the 70 kilodalton σ factor, which is now known to be required for correct promoter recognition. This factor dissociates shortly after initiation of transcription, so it is hardly surprising that it was lost in early purification procedures in which the assays for activity were not designed to score for correct initiation. Another small protein factor called ω (not to be confused with the Type I topoisomerase of *E. coli* also called ω) co-purifies with the so-called holoenzyme, but no functional activity has been demonstrated for this subunit. Other factors have been described which are believed to be required for the initiation or termination of transcription of certain gene products. The current description of the holoenzyme then is that of a pentamer containing σ, 2α, 1 β, and 1 β′, but not necessarily excluding other more or less firmly bound proteins which may be required in some or all transcriptional events.

III. LOCATIONS OF THE GENES FOR RNA POLYMERASE

The genes for the subunits of the holoenzyme are located in three widely dispersed locations on the *E. coli* chromosome; the genes for β and β′ are located adjacent to one another on the same operon. This is not surprising since only β and β′ are required in equimolar amounts to make functional enzyme. Twice as much α is required and, since σ dissociates soon after initiation, it seems likely that less than an equimolar amount of σ is required for optimum utilization of available RNA polymerase. What is surprising, at least initially, is that the genes of the α and β and β′ subunits are parts of large complex operons which also encode some of the genes for ribosomal proteins. The operons which encode the genes for the α and the β and β′ subunits will be referred to as the α and β operons, respectively. It seems likely that the occurrence of ribosomal protein genes and RNA polymerase genes is a device to regulate expression of these genes coordinately. Cells growing with a doubling time of 30 min have about 10 times more ribosomes than polymerases. Clearly, under some conditions, one might expect the synthesis of RNA and protein and the synthesis of the machinery for carrying out these syntheses to be regulated coordinately. It also seems likely that there might be other conditions of growth where the needs for ribosomal proteins and RNA polymerase might not be in the same proportions. A closer look at the β operon, which has been intensively investigated from the standpoint of structure and function, sheds considerable light on this matter.

IV. DETAILED TRANSCRIPTION PATTERN OF THE β OPERON

Most of the detailed analysis of β operon expression began with the isolation of the λ*rif* [d]18 transducing phage, which carries the β operon as well as some other genes found in this region of the host chromosome.[2] One approach used to locate the promoters for the β and β′ genes (*rpo*BC) was to determine how much of the flanking DNA must be jointly excised with the segment containing *rpo*BC expression. Different sized segments containing *rpo*BC were cloned into a λ vector and tested for expression in an infected host. The host was UV-irradiated prior to infection to cut down expression of host genes so that the expression of the λ-carried genes could be seen against a low background as radioactively labeled proteins fractionated on an acrylamide gel. This most effectively and widely used technique is commonly called a ''maxi cell'' experiment. The results of this experiment showed that the main promoter for *rpo*BC expression was located somewhere between the *rpl*A and the *rpl*J genes (see Figure 1). Different orientations of the β operon in the λ vector did not affect the outcome of this experiment eliminating the possibility that the result arose by initiation of transcription from a foreign promoter in the λ vector. Somewhat disquieting was the possibility that because protein products were being examined rather than transcripts some artifact of expression might arise from using heavily irradiated host cells. Subsequent observations have for the most part allayed these fears although an intact transcript for the β operon has yet to be demonstrated. Sequence studies have shown that the promoter proximal gene *rpl*J is separated by about 67 bases from the second gene *rpl*L, and the *rpl*L gene is separated from the third gene *rpo*B by about 321 bases.[4,5] Intercistronic regions of this size frequently serve functions other than spacers between translation reading frames. For example, the *rpl*K and *rpl*A coding sequences (two ribosomal proteins encoded by λ*rif* [d]18)

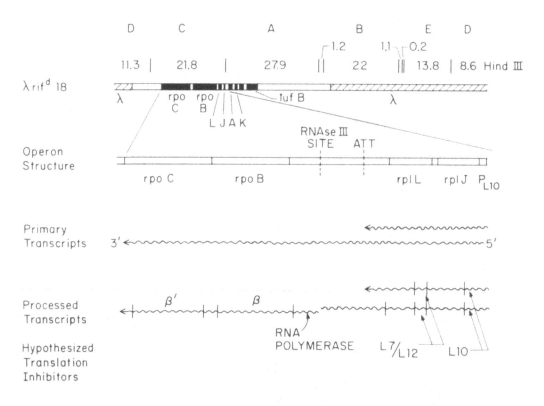

FIGURE 1. Chromosome map of λ*rif* [d]18 and the transcription pattern and hypothesized control mechanisms for β operon expression. L, J, A, K in line 1 indicate *rpl*/L, *rpl*/J, *rpl*/A, and *rpl*/K genes respectively. *rpl*/K and *rpl*/A are transcribed from a promoter (P_{L11}) to the right of K in the diagram. See text for discussion.

are separated by only three base pairs (Figure 1).[5] While it is true that there is a site (P_{L10}) which functions as a promoter of transcription in vitro, it does not follow that this promoter is used in vivo when the upstream sequences are being transcribed from the L11 operon (see Figure 1).[5] Also, possibly significant promoters within the *rpl*J gene[6,7] and between the *rpl*L and *rpo*B genes[8,9] have been described in vitro.

Barry et al.[10] have studied the RNA that originates in vivo from the β operon by hybridization of the total cellular RNA to purified restriction fragments. The hybrids were treated with nuclease S1 to degrade all single-stranded nucleic acid regions and were examined on acrylamide gels. Such studies showed that correctly initiated transcripts frequently terminate at a site about 69 bases downstream from the last codon of the *rpl*L gene (see Figure 1); only about 20% of the transcripts initiated at the β operon promoter (P_{L10}) transcribe beyond this point; these are presumed to be transcribed the full length of the operon. This provisional stop site is termed an attenuator. Comparison of the extended transcripts made in RNAse III[+] and RNAse III[-] strains shows that there is an RNAse III cleavage site 131 bases further downstream from the attenuator. The proposed structures for the attenuator site and the RNAse III cleavage sites are shown in Figure 2. The presence of an attenuator before the *rpo*B gene was first proposed on the basis of the arrangement of the *rpl*JL and *rpo*BC genes[11] and the observation that the ribosomal proteins are present in the cell in greater molar amounts than the RNA polymerase subunits.[12] Differences in translation efficiency could also have accounted for this but the model has now been verified.

Attenuators in λ and *E. coli* biosynthetic operons are modulated by specific regulatory factors. There is some evidence for modulation of the β operon attenuator, but it is not clear by what mechanism this modulation could be carried out.[13] The function of the RNAse III

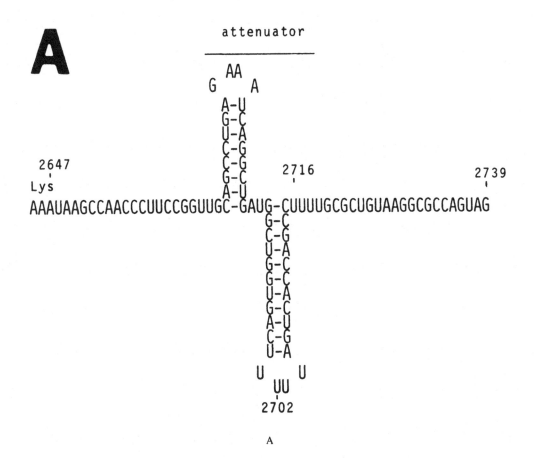

FIGURE 2. RNA sequences within the *rpl*/L-*rpo*B intercistronic region. These sequences are drawn from DNA sequence data presented by Post et al.[5] Numbers indicate the positions in the corresponding DNA sequence. (A) Possible secondary structure near the 3′ end of the attenuated mRNA. (B) RNA sequence in the RNAse III-sensitive region. It is suggested that RNAse III cleaves the double-stranded RNA in the vicinity of position 2860. (From Barry, G., Squires, C., and Squires, C. L., *Proc. Natl. Acad. Sci. U.S.A.*, 77, 3331, 1980.)

cleavage site is even less clear. RNAse III cleavage sites were found in λ and T7 phage messengers and in bacterial ribosomal RNAs but never before in a host messenger.[14] Possibly this "trimming" operation increases the efficiency of translation of the *rpo*BC part of the mRNA by removing RNA which could hinder entering ribosomes. This trimming operation has been shown not to be necessary for translation of most T7 phage messengers.[15] An important exception is the 0.3 protein of T7, the synthesis of which is greatly stimulated both in vivo and in vitro with RNAse III[+] strains. Possibly there is some compensating mechanism which cuts the other mRNAs but which does not cut the mRNA for the 0.3 protein. Alternatively, the other mRNAs do not have to be cut for translation to proceed whereas the mRNA for the 0.3 protein does have to be cut for translation to proceed. A summary of the gross structure of the nascent and processed transcripts believed to be synthesized in vivo from the β operon is given in Figure 1.

V. IN VIVO EVIDENCE THAT THE GENES IN THE β OPERON ARE DIFFERENTIALLY EXPRESSED

The gene arrangement within the β operon and the transcription products suggest several

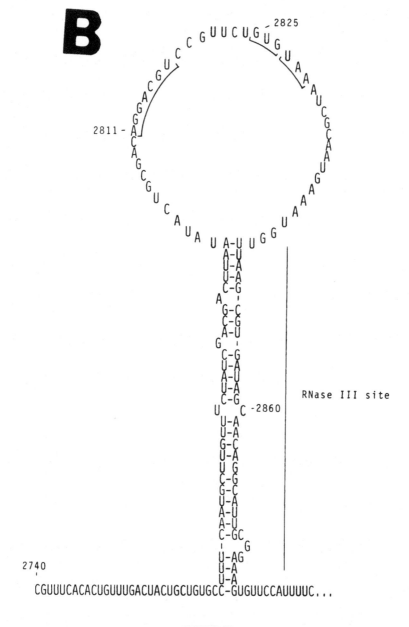

FIGURE 2B.

regulatory modulations such as the attenuator, RNAse processing, and differential translation of the different mRNA units. Observations that the gene products are synthesized in unequal amounts, varying in ratio considerably under different growth conditions, suggest that control of the β operon is complicated. The four gene products L10, L7/12, β, and β' are produced in the molar ratios 1:4:0.2:0.2 under log phase growth conditions.[16-18] However, after instituting stringent growth conditions, which lead to an elevated level of ppGpp,[19] there is a brief period when the synthesis of ribosomal proteins of the β operon is selectively inhibited[12,20] while β and β' are not. Similarly, rifampicin addition to a growing culture inhibits the synthesis of L10 and L7/12 while it produces a transient elevation of ββ' synthesis.[23,24] Streptolydigin, another compound which affects the β subunit and stops both initiation and

Table 1
RELATIVE AMOUNTS OF *rpl*L AND *rpo*BC mRNA MADE IN VITRO[b]

	RNA synthesized		*rpl*L mRNA		*rpo*BC mRNA		Molar ratio (*rpl*L/*rpo*BC
	cpm × 10⁻⁵	Ratio[a]	%	Ratio	%	Ratio	
Control	6.27	1	1.16	1	1.37	1.00	10.1
+ Holoenzyme	16.1	2.57	1.15	0.999	1.97	1.44	7
+ α₂β complex	6.74	1.07	0.99	0.852	1.51	1.10	7.80
+ Rifampicin	1.18	0.188	2.10	1.82	2.24	1.63	11.2
+ Glycerol	9.42	1.50	1.01	0.876	1.71	1.25	7.09

[a] The "ratio" is given as RNA synthesized in presence of effectors divided by RNA synthesized in the control reaction; the "%" is the percent of total RNA synthesized.

[b] Modified from Kajitani, M., Fukuda, R., and Ishihama, A., *Mol. Gen. Genet.*, 179, 489, 1980.

elongation, leads to no selective stimulation of β or β′ subunits.[23] The observations with rifampicin suggest that a mechanism exists for regulating expression of the genes of the β operon after initiation of transcription under different growth conditions. Feedback inhibition of ribosomal protein synthesis at the translation level has been suggested as a mode of regulation in vitro and in vivo, for several operons containing ribosomal protein genes.[25-28] It is possible that the situation with translation of polymerase genes is similar (see also Chapter 3).

Since both ppGpp and rifampicin are believed to interact directly with RNA polymerase, it occurred to a number of investigators that RNA polymerase itself might inhibit its own synthesis at a posttranscriptional or translational level; rifampicin and ppGpp, by complexing with the RNA polymerase, could counteract this inhibitory action. The involvement of RNA polymerase as a regulator of ββ′ synthesis is supported by observations on a strain with a specific temperature sensitive lethal mutation in the gene for the β′ subunit.[29] The synthesis of ββ′ is selectively stimulated in the mutant at nonpermissive temperatures, but not in wild type cells. Another mutant, defective in the β subunit, did not stimulate ββ′ synthesis at nonpermissive temperature. Neither mutant affected α or σ synthesis. Although the experiments described above support the hypothesis that RNA polymerase regulates the synthesis of ββ′, the effects of altering or limiting the RNA polymerase levels in vivo are far reaching and the indirect effects of perturbing the polymerase might account for the observations. More conclusive evidence that the working hypothesis stated above is correct requires that parallel observations be made in vitro under conditions where indirect effects are minimized.

VI. IN VITRO OBSERVATIONS SHOWING THAT ββ′ SYNTHESIS IS NEGATIVELY REGULATED BY RNA POLYMERASE

It has been shown in vitro using λ*drif*⁺-6 DNA (like λ*rif*ᵈ18 but with most of β′ missing) as template that high levels of RNA polymerase produce a marked decrease in the amount of ββ′ synthesis, while not affecting EFTu.[30] Holoenzyme (but not core enzyme) and the α₂β complex (an obligatory intermediate in RNA polymerase assembly) repressed β synthesis. β or β′ had no effect in these in vitro experiments. The authors postulate that in vivo the β subunit in the α₂β complex might be the inhibitor of ββ′ synthesis. The protein EFTu is not encoded by the β operon, so this observation by itself does not relate activity on promoter proximal and promoter distal genes.

Kajitani et al.[31] have studied the RNAs synthesized from λ*rif*ᵈ18 DNA in an in vitro transcription-translation system under a variety of conditions (Table 1). These results are correlated with studies on proteins made under similar conditions.[30] The RNA was measured by hybridizing ^{3}H-UTP labeled RNA to composite plasmids containing pBR322 vectors and either *rpl*L (L10) or *rpl*L with *rpo*B (β)-*rpo*C(β') DNA on filters. The amounts of labeled RNA hybridizable to these DNAs could then be compared with densitometric recordings of proteins separated on SDS-polyacrylamide gels. The $\alpha_2\beta$ complex caused less than a 10% change from control levels in RNA hybridizable to either L10 or ββ' DNA. The L10 peptides were little affected by the addition of $\alpha_2\beta$ complex while ββ' peptide synthesis was severely inhibited. The addition of holoenzyme to the coupled system reduced the differential rate of ββ' RNA; but holoenzyme had a much greater effect on the reduction of ββ' protein synthesis.

Rifampicin had been shown to stimulate transiently ββ' peptide synthesis both in vivo and in vitro. When low levels of rifampicin (5 ng) were added to the in vitro coupled system with λ*rif*[d]18 DNA both ββ' and L10 RNA synthesis were stimulated by about 50%. L10 protein synthesis is not stimulated by rifampicin. Both L10 and L7/12 (the other ribosomal gene in the operon) seem to be regulated autogenously;[32] presumably, the L10 and/or L7/12 proteins could down-regulate synthesis from the 50% excess RNA at a posttranscriptional level. ββ' peptide synthesis on the other hand, if it is autogenously regulated, could be stimulated by the 50% excess RNA if β and/or β' were effectively removed from the pool by rifampicin. Rifampicin binding to the β subunit could affect its possible regulator site directly or might prevent its assembly into an effective down-regulating unit - i.e., $\alpha_2\beta$ or holoenzyme. As noted above, neither β or β' have an effect on in vitro peptide or RNA synthesis when added exogenously. This in vitro picture does not mesh with the results reported above for mutants in vivo where mutants in the β' subunit led to increased synthesis of ββ' peptides while mutants in the β subunit had no significant effect. Since rifampicin is known to bind to the β subunit[33] one would imagine that the role of this subunit in regulation was being affected by rifampicin.

Other experiments[34] have attempted to duplicate in vivo conditions in a reconstructed cell-free system[35,36] with λ*rif*[d]18 DNA. This cell-free system normally contains about 2μg/mℓ of RNA polymerase. The effect of increasing the levels of RNA polymerase up to 10μg/mℓ on gross peptide synthesis and specific protein synthesis was observed (Figures 3 and 4). A two fold rise of total peptide synthesis was observed with increasing concentrations of polymerase over the range of concentrations studies. Three of the λ*rif*[d]18 encoded proteins were studied quantitatively. These include L7/12, EFTu and β and β'. It is clear from the fluorographs that the ratio of L7/12 to ββ' is much higher in this in vitro system than it is in vivo. It is not clear why this is the case. The amounts of EFTu and L7/12 and the total peptide synthesis were elevated when the level of RNA polymerase present during synthesis was increased, but the level of newly synthesized ββ' was substantially reduced. The differential effect of RNA polymerase on L7/12 and ββ' synthesis suggests a selective inhibitory effect on the latter occurring at some point after initiation of transcription of the β operon. A number of variations of this experiment were done to determine the critical factors affecting the synthesis of β and β'. The ratio of RNA polymerase to DNA seems to be a critical factor. For a given level of RNA polymerase the inhibition was less when higher amounts of DNA template were used. This is likely due to a lowering of available polymerase as a result of binding to DNA.

Rifampicin at 1μg/mℓ inhibits the initiation of all transcription. When rifampicin (1μg/mℓ) was introduced at the beginning of cell-free synthesis in these experiments severe inhibition of the synthesis of all proteins of the β operon resulted. In vivo, as mentioned above, it was shown that introduction of rifampicin in a steady state situation resulted in an inhibition of L7/12 synthesis and a transient stimulation of ββ' synthesis.[23,24] The addition of rifampicin 15 min after the start of cell-free synthesis, when most transcription has ceased, and allowing translation to proceed for another 60 min might more nearly approximate the

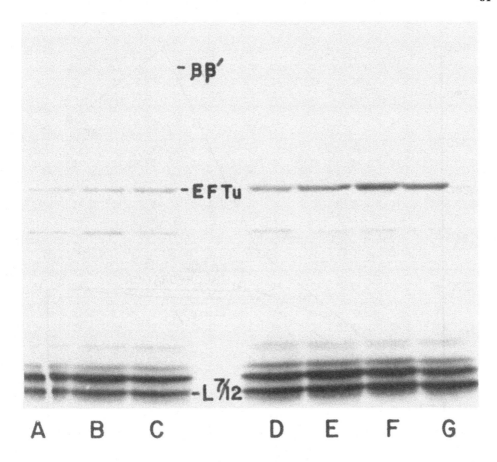

FIGURE 3. Fluorograph of gel electrophoresed ^{3}H-leucine labeled proteins made in a λrif [d]18 DNA-directed coupled system.[32] Positions of ββ', EFTu, and L7/L12 are indicated. In column A the usual reconstructed system was used. In columns B-G increasing levels of purified RNA polymerase (0.5, 1.0, 2.0, 4.0, 6.0, and 8.0 μg/mℓ respectively) were added at the start of synthesis. See text for discussion.

in vivo situation. The effect of rifampicin on ββ' synthesis depended upon the level of RNA polymerase initially present. With no extra RNA polymerase present (about 2μg/mℓ), rifampicin inhibited ββ' synthesis by about 50% (compare columns A and B in Figure 5). When 8μg of RNA polymerase/mℓ was present the amount of ββ' made was reduced to immeasurably low levels (compare columns B and D in Figure 5) unless rifampicin was added (compare columns C and D in Figure 5). The level of inhibition of ββ' synthesis by RNA polymerase varies somewhat between experiments, as can be seen by comparison of the results in Figure 5 with those presented in Figure 3.

This stimulatory effect of rifampicin on ββ' synthesis is interpreted in the following way. At low levels of RNA polymerase, where there is little if any inhibition of ββ' synthesis by RNA polymerase, the effect of adding rifampicin is to block new initiations of transcription, leading to an inhibition of protein synthesis because of the lower level of mRNA synthesis. By contrast, at high levels of RNA polymerase (8μg/mℓ), where ββ' synthesis is severely inhibited, the effect of adding rifampicin is two fold: (1) it inhibits new initiations; and (2) it neutralizes the inhibitory action of high levels of RNA polymerase on ββ' peptide synthesis. The latter effect appears to predominate when rifampicin is added 15 min after starting in vitro synthesis.

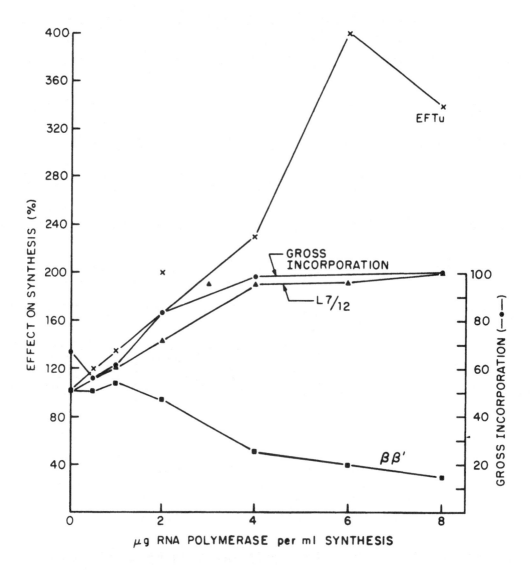

FIGURE 4.   Protein synthesis in the λ*rif* [d]18 DNA-directed coupled system as a function of increasing levels of RNA polymerase. Gross peptide synthesis and the relative amounts of EFTu, ββ', and L7/L12 are indicated. Gross peptide synthesis was estimated by trichloroacetic acid precipitated counts. Amounts of individual proteins were estimated by densitometry of the fluorograph resulting in Figure 3.

VII. SUMMARY

The clustering of genes for RNA polymerase and ribosomal proteins within the same operon provides a means for simultaneously regulating the synthesis of proteins required for transcription and translation. Cells usually have a demand for greater numbers of ribosomes than RNA polymerases - thus the appearance of an attenuator in the β operon between the ribosomal protein genes and the RNA polymerase genes causing premature termination of about 80% of the nascent transcripts. In spite of this coordination at the transcription level there is strong evidence from both in vivo and in vitro observations that β operon encoded proteins are not always coordinately expressed. This evidence comes from experiments where the levels or structures of the proteins in question are appreciably altered as a result of stringent metabolic conditions or the addition of rifampicin.

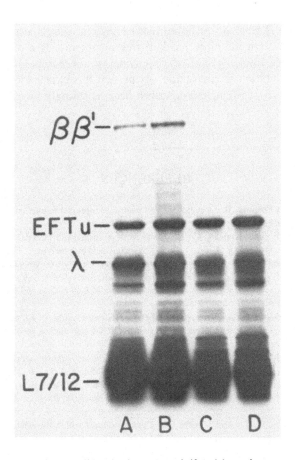

FIGURE 5. Effect of polymerase and rifampicin on the synthesis of the ββ′ subunits. Synthesis was done as described for Figure 3 with the following modifications. In columns A and C 1 μg/mℓ of rifampicin was added 15 min after the start of synthesis and the synthesis was continued for 60 min. In columns C and D, 6 μg/mℓ of additional polymerase was added at the start of synthesis. In arbitrary units the amounts of ββ′ synthesis in A, B, C and D were 63, 114, 22, and 0 respectively. The fluorograph has been overexposed in the EFTu region and below to allow the reliable estimation of ββ′. Lower exposures show that, other than ββ′, rifampicin addition does not stimulate the synthesis of any other proteins detectable in the pattern. The positions of ββ′, EFTu, L7/L12, and an unknown λ protein (labeled λ) are indicated.

In vitro attempts have been made to find conditions where the selective stimulation effect of rifampicin on ββ′ synthesis could be observed and analyzed in greater detail. It has been shown that two conditions must be met to achieve a stimulation effect. When the level of RNA polymerase is high enough to inhibit selectively ββ′ synthesis then the introduction of rifampicin, after the start of cell-free synthesis, leads to a selective stimulatory effect on ββ′ synthesis. Two explanations for this in vitro stimulation are most likely: (1) relief of attenuation leading to more ββ′ mRNA synthesis; or (2) relief of the inhibition by RNA polymerase of ββ′ mRNA translation. The former possibility implies that a high level of polymerase by itself should selectively inhibit *rpo*BC mRNA synthesis, but the preliminary studies described here indicate that this is not the case. Furthermore, the first explanation would require that rifampicin lessen the stalling of polymerase at the attenuator site. This seems unlikely as it is generally believed that rifampicin reacts most effectively with free RNA polymerase.[37-39] On the other hand, if free polymerase is a direct inhibitor of $\beta\beta'$ mRNA translation, the lowering of effective polymerase concentration by rifampicin binding could relieve the inhibition of translation. At present this explanation, at least for the in vitro stimulatory effect of rifampicin described here, is strongly favored.

REFERENCES

1. **Ishihama, A. and Fukuda, R.,** Autogenous and post-transcriptional regulation of RNA polymerase synthesis. *Molecular and Cellular Biochemistry,* 31, 177, 1980.
2. **Kirschbaum, J. B. and Konrad, E. B.,** Isolation of a specialized lambda transducing bacteriophage carrying the β subunit gene for *Escherichia coli* ribonucleic acid polymerase, *J. Bacteriol.,* 116, 517, 1973.
3. **Yamamoto, M. and Nomura, M.,** Cotranscription of genes for RNA polymerase subunits β and β' with genes for ribosomal proteins in *Escherichia coli, Proc. Natl. Acad. Sci. U.S.A.,* 75, 3891, 1978.
4. **Linn, T. and Scaife, J.,** Identification of a single promoter in *Escherichia coli* for *rpl*J, *rpl*L, and *rpo*BC, *Nature,* 276, 33, 1978.
5. **Post, L. E., Strycharz, G. D., Nomura, M., Lewis, H., and Dennis, P. P.,** Nucleotide sequence of the ribosomal protein gene cluster adjacent to the gene for RNA polymerase subunit β in *Escherichia coli, Proc. Natl. Acad. Sci. U.S.A.,* 76, 1697, 1979.
6. **Goldberg, G., Caldwell, P., Weissbach, H., and Brot, N.,***In vitro* regulation of DNA-dependent synthesis of *Escherichia coli* ribosomal protein L12, *Proc. Natl. Acad. Sci. U.S.A.,* 76, 1716, 1979.
7. **Goldberg, G., Zarucki-Schulz, T., Caldwell, P., Weissbach, H., and Brot, N.,** Regulation of the *in vitro* synthesis of *Escherichia coli* ribosomal protein L12, *Biochem. Biophys. Res. Commun.,* 91, 1453, 1979.
8. **Barry, G., Squires, C. L., and Squires, C.,** Control features within the *rpl*JL-*rpo*BC transcription unit of *Escherichia coli, Proc. Natl. Acad. Sci. U.S.A.,* 76, 4922, 1979.
9. **Friesen, J. D., Fiil, N. P., Dennis, P. P., Downing, W. L., An, G., and Holowachuk, E.,** Biosynthetic regulation of *rpl*J, *rpl*L, *rpo*B and *rpo*C in *Escherichia coli,* in *Ribosomes: Structure, Function and Genetics,* Chambliss, G., Craven, G. R., Davies, J., Davis, K., Kahan, L., and Nomura, M., Eds., University Park Press, Baltimore, Md., 1980, 719.
10. **Barry, G., Squires, C., and Squires, C. L.,** Attenuation and processing of RNA from the *rpl*JL-*rpo*BC transcription unit of *Escherichia coli, Proc. Natl. Acad. Sci. U.S.A.,* 77, 3331, 1980.
11. **Lindahl, L., Yamamoto, M., Nomura, M., Kirschbaum, J. B., Allet, B., and Rochaix, J. D.,** Mapping of a cluster of genes for components of the transcriptional and translational machineries of *Escherichia coli, J. Mol. Biol.,* 109, 23, 1977.
12. **Dennis, P. P. and Nomura, M.,** Stringent control of ribosomal protein gene expression in *Escherichia coli, Proc. Natl. Acad. Sci. U.S.A.,* 71, 3819, 1974.
13. **Little, R. and Dennis, P. P.,** Regulation of RNA polymerase synthesis, *J. Biol. Chem.,* 255, 3536, 1980.
14. **Nikolaev, N., Silengo, L., and Schlessinger, D.,** A role for ribonuclease III processing of ribosomal ribonucleic acid and messenger ribonucleic acid precursors in *Escherichia coli, J. Biol. Chem.,* 248, 7967, 1973.
15. **Dunn, J. J. and Studier, F. W.,** Effect of RNAase III cleavage on translation of bacteriophage T7 messenger RNAs, *J. Mol. Biol.,* 99, 487, 1975.
16. **Subramanian, A. R.,** Copies of proteins L7 and L12 and heterogeneity of the large subunit of *Escherichia coli* ribosomes, *J. Mol. Biol.,* 95, 1, 1975.
17. **Dalbow, D. G.,** Synthesis of RNA polymerase in *Escherichia coli* B/r growing at different rates, *J. Mol. Biol.,* 75, 181, 1973.
18. **Matzura, H., Hansen, B. S., and Zeuthen, J.,** Biosynthesis of the β and β' subunits of RNA polymerase in *Escherichia coli, J. Mol. Biol.,* 74, 9, 1973.
19. **Cashel, M. and Gallant, J.,** Two compounds implicated in the function of the RC gene of *Escherichia coli, Nature,* 221, 838, 1969.
20. **Reeh, S., Pedersen, S., and Friesen, J. D.,** Biosynthetic regulation of individual proteins in *rel*A⁺ and *rel*A strains of *Escherichia coli* during amino acid starvation, *Mol. Gen. Genet.,* 149, 279, 1976.

21. **Maher, D. L. and Dennis, P. P.,** *In vivo* transcription of *E. coli* genes coding for rRNA, ribosomal proteins and subunits of RNA polymerase: influence of the stringent control system, *Mol. Gen. Genet.,* 211, 203, 1977.

22. **Blumenthal, R. M., Lemaux, P. G., Neidhardt, F. C., and Dennis, P. P.,** The effects of the *relA* gene on the synthesis of aminoacyl-tRNA synthetases and other transcription and translation proteins in *Escherichia coli* B, *Mol. Gen. Genet.,* 149, 291, 1976.

23. **Nakamura, Y. and Yura, T.,** Effects of rifampicin on synthesis and functional activity of DNA-dependent RNA polymerase in *Escherichia coli, Mol. Gen. Genet.,* 145, 227, 1976.

24. **Hayward, R. S. and Fyfe, S. K.,** Non-coordinate expression of the neighboring genes *rpl*L and *rpo*B,C of *Escherichia coli, Mol. Gen. Genet.,* 160, 77, 1978.

25. **Dean, D. and Nomura, M.,** Feedback regulation of ribosomal protein expression in *Escherichia coli, Proc. Natl. Acad. Sci. U.S.A.,* 77, 3590, 1980.

26. **Fiil, N. P., Friesen, J. D., Downing, W. L., and Dennis, P. P.,** Post-transcriptional regulatory mutants in a ribosomal protein-RNA polymerase operon of *Escherichia coli, Cell,* 19, 837, 1980.

27. **Yates, J. L., Arfsten, A. E., and Nomura, M.,** *In vitro* expression of *Escherichia coli* ribosomal protein genes: autogenous inhibition of translation, *Proc. Natl. Acad. Sci. U.S.A.,* 77, 1837, 1980.

28. **Nomura, M., Morgan, E. A., and Jaskunas, S. R.,** Genetics of bacterial ribosomes, *Ann. Rev. Genet.,* 11, 297, 1977.

29. **Taketo, M. and Ishihama, A.,** Altered synthesis and stability of RNA polymerase holoenzyme subunits in mutants of *Escherichia coli* with mutations in the β or β' subunit genes, *Mol. Gen. Genet.,* 147, 139, 1976.

30. **Fukuda, R., Taketo, M., and Ishihama, A.,** Autogenous regulation of RNA polymerase β subunit synthesis *in vitro, J. Biol. Chem.,* 253, 4501, 1978.

31. **Kajitani, M., Fukuda, R., and Ishihama, A.,** Autogenous and post-transcriptional regulation of *Escherichia coli* RNA polymerase synthesis *in vitro, Mol. Gen. Genet.,* 179, 489, 1980.

32. **Fukuda, R.,** Autogenous regulation of the synthesis of ribosomal proteins L10 and L7/12 in *Escherichia coli, Mol. Gen. Genet.,* 178, 483, 1980.

33. **Zillig, W., Zechel, K., Rabussay, D., Schachner, M., Sethi, V. S., Palm, P., Heil, A., and Seifert, W.,** On the role of different subunits of DNA-dependent RNA polymerase from *E. coli* in the transcription process, *Cold Spring Harbor Symp. Quant. Biol.,* 35, 47, 1970.

34. **Yang, H. L. and Zubay, G.,** Negative regulation of β and β' synthesis by RNA polymerase, *Mol. Gen. Genet.,* 183, 514, 1981.

35. **Zubay, G.,** *In vitro* synthesis of protein in microbial systems, *Ann. Rev. Genet.,* 7, 276, 1974.

36. **Yang, H.-L., Ivashkiv, L., Chen, H-Z., Zubay, G., and Cashel, M.,** A cell-free coupled transcription translation system for investigation of linear DNA segments, *Proc. Natl. Acad. Sci. U.S.A.,* 77, 7029, 1980.

37. **Bahr, W., Stender, W., Scheit, K.-H., and Jovin, T. M.,** Binding of rifampicin to *Escherichia coli* RNA polymerase: thermodynamic and kinetic studies, in *RNA Polymerase,* Losick, R. and Chamberlin, M., Eds., Cold Spring Harbor Monograph Series, 1976, 369.

38. **Wherli, W., Handschin, J., and Wunderli, W.,** Interaction between rifampicin and DNA-dependent RNA polymerase of *Escherichia coli,* in *RNA Polymerase,* Losick, R. and Chamberlin, M., Eds., Cold Spring Harbor Monograph Series, 1976, 397.

39. **Reiness, G., Yang, H.-L., Zubay, G., and Cashel, M.,** Effects of guanosine tetraphosphate on cell-free synthesis of *Escherichia coli* ribosomal RNA and other gene products, *Proc. Natl. Acad. Sci. U.S.A.,* 72, 2881, 1975.

Chapter 6

THE *putA* GENE PRODUCT: TWO ENZYMATIC ACTIVITIES AND A REGULATORY FUNCTION IN A SINGLE POLYPEPTIDE

Rolf Menzel

TABLE OF CONTENTS

I. INTRODUCTION

In *Salmonella typhimurium,* as in several other microorganisms, proline can be utilized as a carbon and nitrogen source. The proteins required for proline catabolism, namely, proline permease, proline oxidase, and △-pyrroline-5-carboxylic acid (PCA) dehydrogenase, are induced by proline and subject to catabolite repression. Both genetic and biochemical analysis of this system in *S. typhimurium* indicate that proline oxidase and PCA dehydrogenase activities are found in a single polypeptide. This protein is the product of the *putA* gene which is located at minute 22 of the *S. typhimurium* genetic map,[7] and is contiguous with *putP* which encodes the cell's major proline permease.[8] The *putA* gene product is a most interesting multifunctional protein that possesses complex catalytic, binding and regulatory activities. First, the two-step oxidation of proline to glutamic acid is shown in Figure 1. The first step, catalyzed by proline oxidase, involves the removal of two electrons from the carbon and nitrogen at positions 1 and 2 of the proline ring with the formation of a double bond.[1,2] In vivo this oxidation is coupled to an electron transport chain which utilizes oxygen as a terminal electron acceptor.[3] The product of this oxidation, pyrroline-5-carboxylic acid (PCA), is in equilibrium γ-glutamic semialdehyde via reversible Schiff's base reaction.[4] PCA may be further oxidized to glutamic acid by PCA dehydrogenase in an NAD[+] dependent reaction.[5] Second, since the enzyme reaction is coupled to electron transport, the *putA* gene product is expected to be associated with the bacterial membrane. This has been found to be the case. Finally, recent genetic evidence implicates this multifunctional protein in regulating the expression of both *putA* and *putP*.[9] This autogenous control of *putA* appears to be independent of its catalytic activities. In the following text, the biochemical evidence for the bifunctional catalytic nature of the *putA* gene product is reviewed and the genetic evidence for autogenous control is discussed.

II. PROPERTIES OF THE *putA* GENE PRODUCT

It has been known for some time that both proline oxidase and PCA dehydrogenase activities are associated with the particulate fraction in extracts of *Escherichia coli.* Based on these observations, Frank and Ranhand[9] have proposed the existence of a "proline oxidation complex." The nature of the proline oxidase activity would require an association with the membrane since in this reaction electrons are transferred to an electron transport chain with oxygen as the terminal electron acceptor.[3] Because there is no such requirement for the PCA dehydrogenase reaction, its particulate nature seems more than coincidental.

Proline utilization has been studied in greater detail in *Salmonella typhimurium.* Ratzkin et al.[7] have analyzed mutants of *S. typhimurium* defective for the oxidation of proline to glutamate. These mutations define the *putA* gene, and in most cases, cause defects in both proline oxidase and PCA dehydrogenase activities. From these results, it can be inferred that an intimate association exists between these two enzymatic activities. Subsequently, Menzel and Roth[6] have found these enzymatic activities in the particulate membrane fraction of disrupted cells. Further, it was shown that both proline oxidase and PCA dehydrogenase could be readily solubilized from the particulate fraction by the use of nonionic detergents. However, in the soluble form, the proline oxidase reaction becomes dependent on an artificial electron acceptor. Both proline oxdase and PCA dehydrogenase activities are enhanced 12-fold following extraction with the detergent. This partially purified preparation was analyzed on native polyacrylamide gels; both proline oxidase and PCA dehydrogenase activities are found in two different species designated Form I and Form II (Figure 2).

When extracts from a *putA* deletion mutant are analyzed in a similar experiment, neither Form I nor Form II are present. Such a deletion extract does show the same substrate-independent reduction bands present in the control gels of the wild type extracts. Molecular

PROLINE OXIDASE

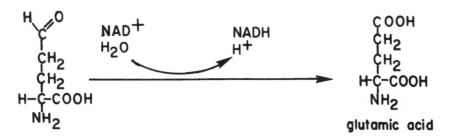

Proline → **Pyrroline-5-carboxylic acid (PCA)** + 2H·

NONENZYMATIC

± H₂O

γ-glutamic acid semialdehyde

PCA DEHYDROGENASE

NAD⁺ + H₂O → NADH + H⁺

glutamic acid

FIGURE 1. Pathway for the oxidation of proline to glutamic acid.

weight estimates were made according to the method of Hedrick and Smyth[10] by running a series of gels similar to that in Figure 2 at different acrylamide concentrations. Molecular weight assignments of 210,000 to 270,000 daltons and 135,000 to 160,000 daltons can be made for Forms I and II, respectively.[6]

The *putA* gene product is readily purified from the detergent treated extract by precipitation with ammonium sulfate, desalting on G-50 Sephadex and chromatography on DEAE.[6] Both proline oxidase and PCA dehydrogenase co-purify to near homogeneity in this procedure (Figure 3). It is readily apparent that both enzyme activities are eluted together and coincide with the only protein peak that elutes with the salt gradient. The peak fractions were pooled and analyzed on denaturing SDS gels (Figure 4). Contaminating protein is only observed when the gel is substantially overloaded with sample (3.6 μg, left lane). A densitometer

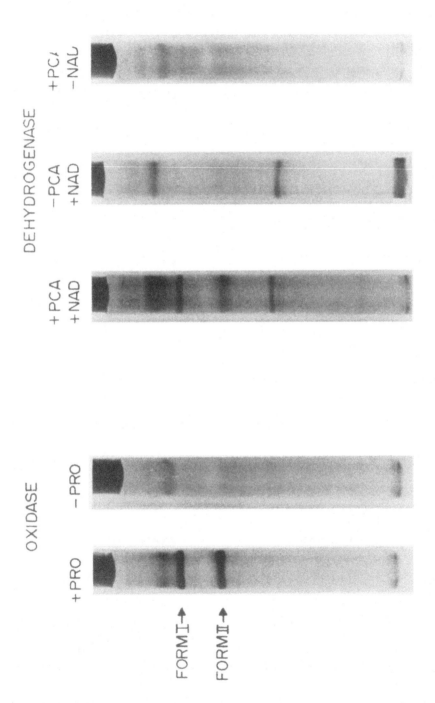

FIGURE 2.   Native gel electrophoresis of Tween 20 extracts of *S. typhimurium* induced for proline oxidase and PCA dehydrogenase activities. Electrophoresis was carried out as described. The gels were stained for both proline oxidase and PCA dehydrogenase. Although nonspecific reactions are apparent (columns marked −pro, −PCA +NAD, +PCA −NAD), two bands are readily observed when all substrates were present. (From Menzel, R. and Roth, J. R., *J. Biol. Chem.*, 256, 9755, 1981. With permission.)

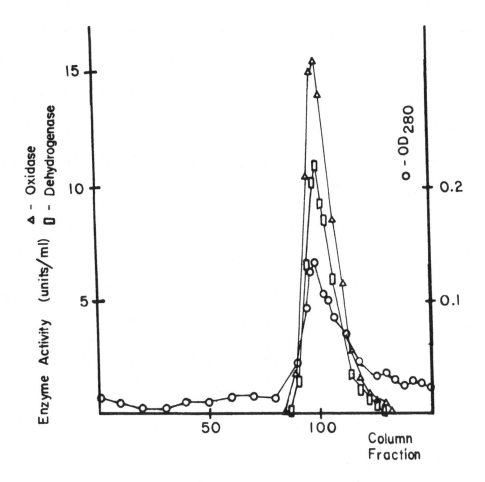

FIGURE 3. Representative profile of a DEAE column used to purify the *putA* gene product. Membrane associated proteins were extracted with Tween 20, precipitated with $(NH_4)_2SO_4$, desalted with G-50 Sephadex and applied to a 100 mℓ DEAE Sephadex A25 column. The protein was eluted with a 60 to 160 m*M* KCl gradient, and proline oxidase (△-△), PCA dehydrogenase (□-□), and (○-○) protein were monitored. Activities are expressed in units/mℓ of column effluent, and protein is expressed as A_{280}. (From Menzel, R. and Roth, J. R., *J. Biol. Chem.*, 256, 9755, 1981. With permission.)

tracing of such gels indicate that 97% of the protein is present as a single band and that none of the contaminating protein account for more than 1% of the protein added to the gel. The mobility of the purified protein was compared to the migration of the molecular weight standards in denaturing gels and a molecular weight of 132,000 daltons was assigned to the purified *putA* gene product.[6] Since two forms of this protein had been previously found (see Figure 2), the molecular weight of the purified protein was determined by nondenaturing gel electrophoresis. Only Form I is purified by this procedure. Since the *putA* gene product is present in two molecular weight forms after the membrane is solubilized with detergent, and since both forms have proline oxidase and PCA dehydrogenase activities, this author concludes that Form II is most likely an active monomer that is lost during purification. Presumably, Form I is an active dimer of the 132,000 dalton peptide. When purified Form I is subjected to velocity sedimentation, it has a size similar to that of catalase (240,000) which agrees very well with the analysis on native gels.

That the 132,000 dalton peptide purified by the procedure outlined above has properties appropriate to that of the *putA* gene product is supported further by the following results:

1.   Proline oxidase is inducible by proline and subject to catabolite repression.[7,11] SDS

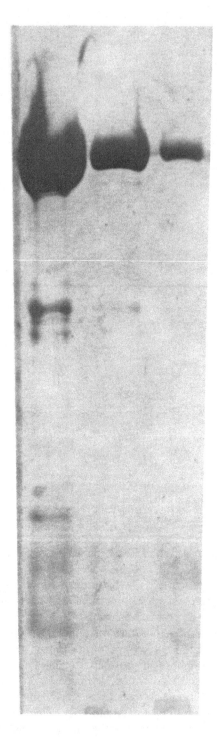

FIGURE 4.   Denaturing gel electrophoresis of the purified *putA* gene product. SDS polyacrylamide electrophoresis was performed as described. The left lane contains 3.6 μg of protein; the center lane, 0.6 μg of protein; the right lane, 0.05 μg of protein. (From Menzel, R. and Roth, J. R., *J. Biol. Chem.*, 256, 9755, 1981. With permission.)

polyacrylamide gels of detergent extracts from wild type cells show that the 132,000 dalton peptide is subject to induction by proline and repression by glucose.[6]

2. The 132,000 dalton peptide is absent in a *putA* amber mutant grown under inducing conditions.[6]

The purification results in the preparation of a protein which is essentially homogeneous following a 52-fold purification. This indicates that the *putA* gene product accounts for approximately 2% of the cell's protein in cells which are fully induced. SDS-polyacrylamide gels of crude extracts verify this conclusion. The *putA* gene product is a major protein in cells that are fully induced.

When cells are made diploid by the introduction of an F-plasmid, it is found that no two *putA* mutations will complement to give a *putA*[+] phenotype. The *putA* mutants define a single complementation group as is expected for a gene encoding a single polypeptide. The *putA* gene has been cloned and *putA* functions (proline oxidase and PCA dehydrogenase) have been localized to a 4.1 kilobase fragment of DNA. Such a fragment has a maximum peptide coding capacity of approximately 150,000 daltons. Minicells containing the above plasmid produce the 132,000 dalton peptide believed to be the *putA* gene product.[17]

The proline oxidase and PCA dehydrogenase activities of the purified *putA* gene product are different from one another with respect to optimum reaction conditions, substrate requirements, and reaction mechanisms.[13] The purified *putA* protein is a flavoprotein.[13] The flavin group is involved in proline oxidase, but not PCA dehydrogenase. The purified *putA* protein, thus, catalyzes two distinct enzymatic reactions required for the oxidation of proline to glutamic acid.

III. GENETIC ANALYSIS OF THE *putA* GENE

The *putA* gene is part of a two-gene cluster which encodes functions necessary for proline utilization.[7] The second gene, *putP*, encodes the cell's major proline permease.[8] This two-gene cluster maps at minute 22 of the *S. typhimurium* genetic map.[14] The gene cluster is defined by a series of point and deletion mutations. The genetic map shown in Figure 5 has been generated as follows. Phage P22 was propagated on *S. typhimurium* containing point mutations in *putA* or *putP* and used to transduce recipient strains containing deletions of the *putA-putP* region. The map shows a border separating the *putA* gene from the *putP* gene drawn between mutations *838* and *741*. The mutation *741* and all those to the right of it (except *900*, discussed below) are defective for the enzymatic activities required to oxidize proline to glutamate and define the *putA* gene. The mutation *838* and all those to the left of it are defective for the cell's major proline permease and define the *putP* gene. The permease negative phenotype may be determined by resistance to the proline analogue azetidine carboxylic acid (AZT[R]) or by measuring proline transport directly.[8]

A striking feature of the genetic analysis is that strains harboring insertion mutations are defective in either *putA* or *putP*. No insertion mutation leads to the double mutant phenotype of *putA*[-] and *putP*[-]. Lack of polarity for insertion mutants (as well as some examples of amber mutants) implies the *putA* and *putP* genes are transcribed independently. Nevertheless, these two genes are physically very close to one another. Co-transductional frequencies for mutations near the gene border are very high; >95%.[7] Small deletions (e.g., *put557*) which remove both *putA* and *putP* functions have no other detectable phenotype. Sequence analysis of cloned DNA from the gene border indicates the region is on the order of 500 base pairs and contains promoters for both *putA* and *putP*.[17]

Mutations that affect the enzyme activities of the *putA* gene product show two phenotypes with respect to the regulation of the *putP* gene. Wild type cells are sensitive to the proline analogue azetidine carboxylic acid (AZT[S]). Mutants defective for the *putP* gene are resistant

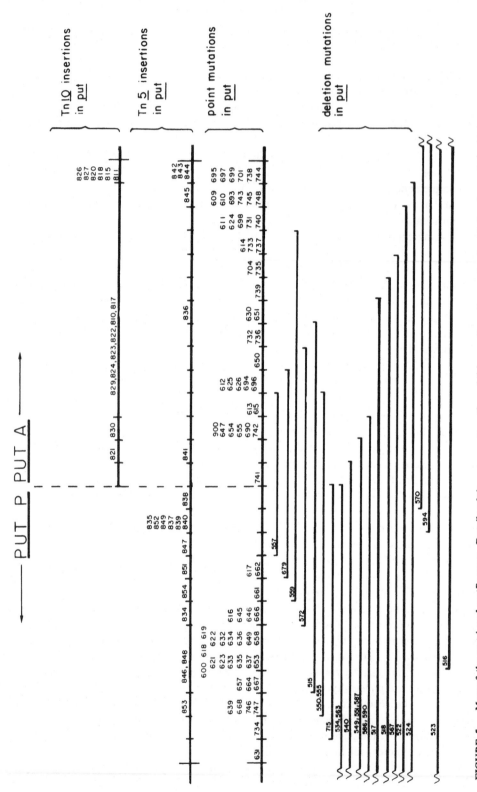

FIGURE 5. Map of the *putA* and *putP* genes. Details of the map construction of this genetic region can be found elsewhere. (From Menzel, R. and Roth, J. R., *J. Mol. Biol.*, 148, 21, 1981. With permission.)

to AZT. Mutants constitutive for both the expression of proline oxidase and proline permease show a heightened sensitivity to AZT (AZT^{SS} phenotype).[12] Mutants lacking proline oxidase activity may be either sensitive to AZT at a level similar to that of wild type cells (AZT^S) or demonstrate a heightened sensitivity (AZT^{SS}) similar to that of mutants constitutive for the expression of the *put* genes. The *putA*$^-$ mutants which are AZT^{SS} were shown to have lost their ability to regulate the permease.[12] They behave like constitutive mutants for the *putP* gene. All insertion and amber mutants in the *putA* gene are in the AZT^{SS} class.

Dendinger and Brill[11] have isolated a mutant constitutive for the expression of both proline oxidase and proline permease. Ratzkin et al.[7] have demonstrated that this mutation, *putA900*, maps at the position indicated in Figure 5. This mutation maps within the *putA* gene between insertion mutations which cause a loss of the enzymatic activities of the *putA* gene. Menzel and Roth[12] have isolated other constitutive mutants and mapped two independent constitutive mutations in the same deletion intervals as *putA* mutants *732* and *609*. Mutants constitutive for the expression of both *putA* and *putP* map throughout the *putA* gene.

The *putA* gene product must also code for a regulatory function in addition to two distinct enzymatic activities. To distinguish the various phenotypes of different *putA* alleles, Menzel and Roth[12] have adopted a nomenclature using the letter "A" to denote enzymatic activities and the letter "C" to denote control function. The wild type is designated A$^+$C$^+$, it has both the enzymatic activities and normal control functions. Mutants defective for the enzymatic activities are A$^-$ and may be either A$^-$C$^+$ (has normal control function) or A$^-$C$^-$ (is defective for regulation and expresses *putP* constitutively). A mutant which is constitutive for proline oxidase is A$^+$C$^-$ (has the enzymatic activities and is defective for control). All mutants constitutive for the expression of proline oxidase are also constitutive for the expression of *putP*.

Some definite predictions can be made about the types of revertants expected for both A$^-$C$^+$ and A$^-$C$^-$ mutations. Alterations in a protein's structure which correct a defect in enzymatic activity may or may not alter the protein's regulatory function. It is expected that most revertants would be to a wild type protein (A$^+$C$^+$) with a minor class retaining or gaining a defect in control functions. For both A$^-$C$^+$ and A$^-$C$^-$ mutants, the major class or revertants were observed to be A$^+$C$^+$.[12] Among certain A$^-$C$^+$ and A$^-$C$^-$ mutants, a minor class of A$^+$C$^-$ revertants were seen. The reversion events of the class A$^-$C$^-$ reverting to A$^+$C$^+$ (a common event) and A$^-$C$^+$ reverting to A$^+$C$^-$ (a rare event) demonstrate the simultaneous mutation of two phenotypes, enzyme activity and control function, while selection was made for only a single phenotype, enzyme activity.

When a diploid is constructed (using an F$'$ plasmid) with both a constitutive A$^+$C$^-$ mutation and a wild type allele of the *putA* gene, the resultant strain shows normal regulation.[12] The constitutive phenotype is, therefore, recessive. The *putA* A$^-$C$^+$ mutant type is also able to correct the regulatory defect of the *putA* A$^+$C$^-$ constitutive mutant in trans. The *putA* A$^-$C$^-$ mutant type is unable to complement the constitutive. The assignment of the presence or absence of control function in A$^-$ mutants based on the regulation of the permease is confirmed by complementation tests with constitutive A$^+$C$^-$ mutants.

The properties of the wild type and three different mutant types of the *putA* gene are summarized in Table 1. All insertion mutations and amber mutations lead to the A$^-$C$^-$ phenotype. Loss of the *putA* gene product results in the loss of both enzyme activity and control functions. Efforts to identify insertion mutations which lead to the constitutive phenotype have failed.[12] Analysis of mutants with the A$^-$C$^+$ phenotype suggest they are missense mutants.[12] It seems likely that the missense mutations can lead to the loss of either enzyme activities or control activity without loss of the second aspect of *putA* function (the A$^-$C$^+$ and A$^+$C$^-$ mutant types).

The mechanism by which the *putA* gene product exerts its control function is not known. Complementation tests have shown that a regulatory defect can be corrected in trans for

Table 1
A SUMMARY OF THE VARIOUS MUTANT PHENOTYPES OF THE *putA* GENE

Mutant type	Enzymatic activity	Permease regulation	Ability to repress a constitutive mutation present in trans
A⁺ C⁺ (wild type)	Yes	Yes	Yes
A⁺ C⁻ (constitutive mutant)	Yes	No	No
A⁻ C⁺	No	Yes	Yes
A⁻ C⁻	No	No	No

putA A^+C^- mutants. Such trans correction is consistent with a repressor type control system.[15,16] The most direct model would propose that the *putA* gene product acts as a repressor of both its own synthesis and that of the adjacent *putP* gene. The failure to detect any additional genes involved in control supports such a direct repressor model of control. Such a failure is not definitive and additional experiments are underway in an effort to demonstrate repressor type interactions between purified *putA* protein and *put* DNA. Although the *putA* gene product will bind DNA it fails to show specificity for *put* DNA.[17] Regardless of the mechanism by which the *putA* gene exerts its control function, it is clear that the control function is independent of the degradative enzyme activities. Mutants defective for enzyme activities may (A^-C^+) or may not (A^-C^-) possess regulatory activity.

IV. CONCLUSIONS

Any autogenously controlled system should have the range of mutant types and reversion patterns seen for the *putA* gene. For the gene of an autogenously controlled enzyme, there should be missense mutations which affect either regulatory function or catalytic activity alone. Mutations which result in the complete loss of gene product will have the double mutant phenotype. When the regulatory function is postulated to be a repressor-type control function then missense mutations may or may not complement a constitutive mutation. The reversion of mutations defective for enzymatic activity may uncover mutations which have lost regulatory functions.

A speculative model can provide a rationale for a membrane-bound protein which represses its own synthesis. The oxidase reaction of the *putA* gene product is dependent on the presence of a membrane-bound electron transport chain which uses oxygen as its terminal electron acceptor. For the *putA* gene product to become functional it must interact with an electron transport chain. Menzel and Roth[12] have postulated that there are membrane sites with which the *putA* protein must interact to become functional. Upon induction (exposure to proline containing media), the *putA* gene product is synthesized and inserted into functional membrane sites. Once such functional sites have been "titrated", excess *putA* gene product (not membrane-bound) may act as a repressor of the *put* genes. Whether the *putA* gene products' regulation proceeds by a "titration of functional sites" is not yet clear and will require further analysis.

The concept of "titration of functional sites" finds a precedent in the case of the gene 32 product of phage T4 discussed in this book. T4 gene 32 product is a single-stranded DNA binding protein which is autogenously controlled. In the model of the regulation of T4 gene 32 product, Doherty and co-workers (see Chapter 4) propose that gene 32 product is synthesized until all the single-stranded DNA binding sites are titrated. At this point the excess gene 32 product binds to its own message turning off the synthesis of more gene 32 production at the translation level. The work of Yates and co-workers (see Chapter 3) also discussed in this book demonstrates that a number of ribosomal proteins are autogenously controlled. Regulation of these proteins can be seen in the "titration of functional sites" paradigm if the assembling ribosome is considered the 'site' to be titrated. The notion of "titration of functional sites" may be a useful paradigm which might apply to a number of autogenously controlled systems.

ACKNOWLEDGMENTS

The large majority of this work represents the author's doctoral thesis for the Molecular Biology Department of the University of California at Berkeley. The cloning and sequence analysis mentioned in this text was done at the Howard Hughes Medical Institute in the Biology Department of the University of Utah.

REFERENCES

1. **Strecker, H. J. and Mela, P.,** The interconversion of glutamic acid and proline, *Biochim. Biophys. Acta,* 17, 580, 1955.
2. **Strecker, H. J.,** The interconversion of glutamic acid and proline II. The preparation and properties of Δ'-pyrroline-5-carboxylic acid, *J. Biol. Chem.,* 235, 2045, 1960.
3. **Strecker, H. J.,** The preparation of animal proline oxidase (rat liver), and its use for the preparation of Δ'-pyrroline-5-carboxyate, *Methods Enzymol.,* 17B, 251, 1971.
4. **Vogel, H. J. and David, B.,** Glutamic γ-semialdehyde and Δ'-pyrroline-5-carboxylic acid, intermediates in the biosynthesis of proline, *J. Am. Chem. Soc.,* 74, 109, 195.
5. **Stretcker, H. J.,** The interconversion of glutamic acid and proline III. Δ'-pyrroline-5-carboxylic acid dehydrogenase, *J. Biol. Chem.,* 235, 3218, 1960.
6. **Menzel, R. and Roth, J. R.,** Purification of the *putA* gene product: a bifunctional membrane-bound protein from *Salmonella typhimurium* responsible for the two-step oxidation of proline to glutamate, *J. Biol. Chem.,* 256, 9755, 1981.
7. **Ratzkin, B., Grabnar, M., and Roth, J. R.,** Regulation of the major proline permease gene of *Salmonella typhimurium, J. Bacteriol.,* 133, 737, 1978.
8. **Ratzkin, B. and Roth, J. R.,** Cluster of genes controlling proline degradation in *Salmonella typhimurium, J. Bacteriol.,* 133, 744, 1978.
9. **Frank, L. and Ranhand, B.,** Proline metabolism in *Escherichia coli.* III. The proline catabolic pathway, *Arch. Biochem. Biophys.,* 107, 325, 1964.
10. **Hedrick, J. L. and Smyth, A. J.,** Size and charge isomer separation and estimation of molecular weights of proteins by disc gel electrophoresis, *Arch. Biochem. Biophys.,* 126, 155, 1968.
11. **Dendinger, S. and Brill, W. J.,** Regulation of proline degradation in *Salmonella typhimurium, J. Bacteriol.,* 103, 144, 1970.
12. **Menzel, R. and Roth, J. R.,** Regulation of the genes for proline utilization in *Salmonella typhimurium*: autogenous repression by the *putA* product, *J. Mol. Biol.,* 148, 21, 1981.
13. **Menzel, R. and Roth, J. R.,** Enzymatic properties of the purified *putA* protein from *Salmonella typhimurium, J. Biol. Chem.,* 256, 9762, 1981.
14. **Sanderson, K. E. and Hartman, P. E.,** Linkage map of *Salmonella typhimurium, Microbiol. Rev.,* 42, 471, 1978.
15. **Jacob, F. and Monod, J.,** Genetic regulatory mechanism in the synthesis of proteins, *J. Mol. Biol.,* 3, 318, 1961.
16. **Epstein, B. and Beckwith, J.,** Regulation of gene expression, *Annu. Rev. Biochem.,* 37, 411, 1968.
17. **Menzel, R.,** manuscript being prepared.

Chapter 7

CONSIDERATION OF GLUTAMINE SYNTHETASE AS A MULTIFUNCTIONAL PROTEIN

Jean E. Brenchley

TABLE OF CONTENTS

I. INTRODUCTION

The amino acid glutamine is not only essential for protein synthesis but also as a precursor for other nitrogen-containing compounds in cells. The enzyme responsible for glutamine production, glutamine synthetase, is widely distributed in microorganisms, plants, and animals and catalyzes the conversion of glutamate and ammonia to glutamine with the cleavage of ATP to ADP and P_i. Glutamine synthetase occupies a central position in cell physiology, because it forms an intersection of pathways for carbon metabolism, ammonia assimilation, amino acid synthesis, and the availability of glutamate and glutamine as precursors for other cell constituents. Many microorganisms use glutamate synthase, which converts glutamine and α-ketoglutarate to two glutamates, as the primary route for glutamate production. For these organisms, glutamine synthetase has the interesting physiological role of using glutamate as a substrate to make glutamine, which serves as a product for other cell metabolism and as a precursor for producing more glutamate. In this role, glutamine synthetase is in a cyclic reaction necessary for making one of its substrates.

Because of its central role in metabolism, there has been considerable interest in the structure, catalytic sites, and regulation of glutamine synthetases from a variety of organisms and tissues since the first studies of glutamine metabolism by Krebs in 1935.[1] This interest is reflected by the publication of two books covering the broad topic of glutamine metabolism.[2,3] A review of this vast amount of information on different glutamine synthetases from different microorganisms, animals, and plants is beyond the scope of this article. In order to focus on the topic of glutamine synthetase as a multifunctional protein, this chapter will be limited to studies with microorganisms where genetic and biochemical information have been combined to examine glutamine synthetase as an enzyme with the possible function as a regulator of protein synthesis. This criterion limits the article to a primary consideration of work with the enteric bacteria. The first stage of the article will briefly outline some of the interesting biochemical features of glutamine synthetase from these organisms. The second phase will summarize the early results suggesting that glutamine synthetase has a function in regulation; and the third will survey recent information identifying other components involved in regulating synthesis of glutamine synthetase and other enzymes involved in nitrogen utilization.

II. CATALYTIC ACTIVITY OF GLUTAMINE SYNTHETASE

The glutamine synthetase from *Escherichia coli* has been extensively studied and the information reviewed.[4-7] Although there are properties that differ for the glutamine synthetases from *E. coli*, *Salmonella typhimurium*, *Klebsiella aerogenes*, and *K. pneumoniae*, the characteristics described for the enzyme from *E. coli* are generally applicable to these proteins.[8] The enzyme has a molecular weight of 600,000 daltons and is composed of 12 identical subunits with a molecular weight of about 50,000 daltons each. Electron micrographs of purified glutamine synthetase show that the subunits are arranged in a hexagonal bilayer with a layer of six subunits superimposed on the other.[6,9] These bilayered molecules can polymerize face to face, to form long strands which wind around each other to form three- and seven-stranded cables.[10,11]

In addition to its normal biosynthetic activity (Reaction 1), glutamine synthetase can catalyze a γ-glutamyl transfer reaction (Reaction 2) where, in the presence of ADP, divalent metal ions, and arsenate, the γ-glutamyl moiety of glutamine is transferred to hydroxylamine, and γ-glutamyl hydroxamate is formed. This γ-glutamyl transfer reaction is a catalytic activity of the enzyme and has been particularly useful as an assay for glutamine synthetase.[4]

Reaction 1:

$$\text{L-glutamate} + \text{ATP} + \text{NH}_4^+ \xrightarrow{\text{(divalent metal ion)}}$$

$$\text{L-glutamine} + \text{ADP} + \text{P}_i$$

Reaction 2:

$$\text{L-glutamine} + \text{NH}_2\text{OH} \xrightarrow[\text{ADP} + \text{arsenate}]{\text{(divalent metal ion)}}$$

$$\gamma\text{-glutamylhydroxamate} + \text{NH}_4^+$$

The reaction mechanism for glutamine synthesis appears to occur by the formation of enzyme-bound intermediates, including γ-glutamyl phosphate.[6,7] Evidence for the formation of the phosphorylated intermediate comes from several studies with analogs. One example is the use of L-methionine-SR-sulfoximine, a proposed transition-state analog, which is phosphorylated by glutamine synthetase in the presence of ATP and remains bound to the enzyme as the phosphorylated intermediate.[12-15] L-methionine-SR-sulfoximine has been useful in locating the substrate binding sites. It appears that the oxygen atom of the sulfoximine binds to the site for the carboxyl oxygen atom of glutamate that does not get phosphorylated. The nitrogen atom of the sulfoximine binds at the site for the oxygen atom that is phosphorylated, and the methyl group of the methionine sulfoximine binds the ammonia binding site.[7,14,16-21] This positioning allows the nitrogen atom of the sulfoximine to be phosphorylated.

Recently, mutants of *S. typhimurium* resistant to the growth inhibition of methionine sulfoximine have been isolated and characterized.[22,23] The glutamine synthetase activities from these mutants are resistant to inhibition by methionine sulfoximine, have reduced γ-glutamyl transferase activities and higher apparent Km values for glutamate and ammonia but not for ATP.[23] These results are consistent with a mutation that alters the active site of glutamine synthetase and simultaneously changes the affinities for the L-methionine-SR-sulfoximine, glutamate, and ammonia. The characterization of these and similar mutants should provide a genetic approach for the mapping of substrate binding sites that will augment the information from physical studies.

III. REGULATION OF GLUTAMINE SYNTHETASE ACTIVITY

The activity of glutamine synthetase from the enteric bacteria can be regulated through feedback inhibition by numerous products of glutamine metabolism, by the presence of divalent metal ions, and by covalent modification involving the adenylylation and deadenylylation of a tyrosyl residue on each subunit.[4-6] These reactions are delicately balanced by cell physiology and may have different roles in changing glutamine synthetase activity. The relevant point for this article is the existence of numerous binding sites on each glutamine synthetase subunit that are involved in modulating activity (Figure 1). In addition to the substrate binding sites for glutamate, ATP, and ammonia, there are sites for feedback inhibitors, metal ions, and the modification enzyme, adenyl transferase. It is also clear that the glutamine synthetase proteins can exist in a number of forms within the cell. Since each of the 12 subunits of glutamine synthetase can exist in the deadenylylated or adenylylated state, a number of hybrid proteins consisting of varying degrees of adenylylation from 0 to 12 subunits can exist. These adenylylation states can in turn influence the metal ion requirements, stability, oxidation, and inhibition and the activity of glutamine synthetase.

A consideration of all the variables that influence glutamine synthetase activity quickly illustrates that each subunit must recognize a number of signals. Although some sites for

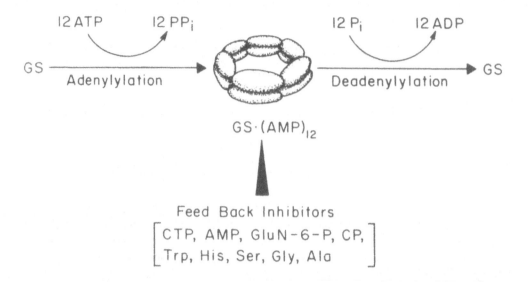

FIGURE 1. Diagram of glutamine synthetase illustrating feedback inhibition and the adenylylation-deadenylylation process. The abbreviations are: GS, deadenylylated glutamine synthetase; GS (AMP)$_{12}$, adenylylated glutamine synthetase; CTP, cytosine triphosphate; AMP, adenosine monophosphate; GluN-6-P, glucosamine 6-phosphate; carbamyl phosphate; Trp, L-tryptophan; His, L-histidine; Ser, L-serine; Gly, glysine; Ala, L-alanine.

binding the feedback inhibitors may be shared, there are separate sites for at least alanine, tryptophan, histidine, AMP, and CTP.[6] In addition to the physical studies examining the relationships of the sites for the substrates, feedback inhibitors, and metals mentioned above, there are some interesting biochemical experiments analyzing the subunit structure relative to the AMP binding site.[24-27] Limited proteolysis of purified glutamine synthetase yields two primary fragments.[26-27] One large fragment of about 35,000 daltons and a smaller fragment of about 15,000 daltons are formed. When [AMP-8-^{14}C] adenylylated glutamine synthetase was treated with limiting subtilisin and the protein fragments observed by electrophoresis in the presence of sodium dodecyl sulfate, the radioactive AMP remained with the 35,000 dalton fragment.[27] These results located the AMP site on the larger fragment obtained with limited digestion of purified glutamine synthetase.[26,27]

Recently, we have sequenced part of the DNA encoding glutamine synthetase from *S. typhimurium* and have determined the location of the tyrosine that is modified by AMP.[28,29] The sequence data show that the AMP site is about 200 nucleotides (or 70 amino acids) from the region encoding the carboxyterminal amino acids. The inferred amino acid sequence of this region shows considerable homology with that determined for the AMP-containing peptide of the *E. coli* protein.[24,29,30] Of an inferred sequence of 35 amino acids, there were four that differed from the sequence determined for the *E. coli* peptide.[29,30] The DNA sequence not only provides information about the region near the tyrosine that is modified by AMP for the protein from *S. typhimurium,* but it also identifies its position in the amino acid sequence. Its location near the carboxyterminal amino acids is interesting, since other studies have shown that the AMP lies on the surface of the subunit.[31,32] One method used to study the AMP binding site has been the preparation of antibodies that will specifically recognize this modification.[32,33] The results of electron micrographs of the antibody-glutamine synthetase complexes localized the AMP site on the outer edge of the hexagonal disc.[32] The combination of the biochemical information identifying the positions of the AMP site in the primary sequence and the physical studies locating the site on the enzyme will help us understand the formation and function of this site on glutamine synthetase.

Even this superficial survey of the biochemical properties illustrates the structural complexity of glutamine synthetase. If one considers the definition of a multifunctional protein as one that structurally consists of a single type of polypeptide chain that has multiple catalytic or binding functions, then the diverse biochemical properties of glutamine synthetase make it a candidate.[34]

The summation of binding sites for metals, substrates, and feedback inhibitors seems extraordinarily large for each 50,000 dalton subunit. Then, in addition, the presence of the AMP modification site adds a dimension not seen with many other proteins. Within the framework of considering glutamine synthetase as a multifunctional protein, the adenylylation process is of particular interest. During the adenylylation and deadenylylation process, glutamine synthetase is, in essence, serving as a substrate for another enzyme reaction. The modification process in turn has a large effect on the conformation of glutamine synthetase and changes the binding of many other effectors. In this regard, glutamine synthetase binds and responds to several effectors, has its own important catalytic activity, and has a site that serves as a substrate for the adenyl transferase enzyme. These aspects alone make glutamine synthetase a complicated multifaceted enzyme, but in addition to these features is the consideration of whether glutamine synthetase can function as a regulator of protein synthesis.

IV. GLUTAMINE SYNTHETASE AS A REGULATOR OF PROTEIN SYNTHESIS

A. Early Evidence for a Regulatory Function

The proposal that glutamine synthetase is involved in the regulation of protein synthesis was based primarily on results with mutants of *K. aerogenes*. This section will review only a few of the critical results that led to this proposal; a more comprehensive review of these earlier investigations is available.[35] The initial work dealt with the regulation of histidine utilization (*hut*) as a nitrogen source by *K. aerogenes*. It had been observed that histidase, the first enzyme for histidine degradation, was produced at higher levels in cells grown in a medium with glucose as a carbon source and histidine as a nitrogen source than in medium with glucose, ammonium, and histidine.[36,37] Histidase activities decreased when a more rapidly utilizable nitrogen source was available and increased when higher activities of histidase were needed to use histidine as a nitrogen source. This response can be referred to as nitrogen control or nitrogen catabolite repression. The implication that glutamine synthetase functioned as a regulatory molecule during nitrogen control came from a number of studies. First, physiological experiments demonstrated that glutamine synthetase activities also increased in cells grown in a medium with a limiting nitrogen source such as histidine (Table 1), and in fact there was a direct correlation between glutamine synthetase and histidase activities for a variety of growth conditions.[38,39] In contrast, the measurement of one of the glutamate synthesizing enzymes, glutamate dehydrogenase, showed that its activity consistently decreased whenever glutamine synthetase activities were high (see Table 1).[40,41] Because a second enzyme, glutamate synthase, exists that can produce glutamate during a nitrogen-limiting growth condition, glutamate dehydrogenase activities were not essential and could be repressed when *K. aerogenes* was growing in these media. Glutamine auxotrophs lacking an active glutamine synthetase were unable to increase histidase levels or reduce glutamate dehydrogenase levels when the cells were limited for a nitrogen source. In contrast, mutants with elevated glutamine synthetase activities also had higher induced levels of histidase and reduced glutamate dehydrogenase activities even when grown in a medium with high concentrations of ammonia.[38-41]

These results simply demonstrated that a correlation existed between the responses for glutamine synthetase, histidase, and glutamate dehydrogenase and did not exclude the possibilities that they shared a common control or that the mutations affecting glutamine syn-

Table 1

**SUMMARY OF MUTATIONS AFFECTING HISTIDASE
REGULATION IN *K. aerogenes*[a]**

Strain	Growth condition	Glutamine synthetase activity	Histidase activity	Glutamate dehydrogenase activity
Gln+	Nitrogen excess	Low	Low	High
Gln+	Nitrogen limited	High	High	Low
Gln−	Nitrogen excess	Absent	Low	High
Gln−	Nitrogen limited	Absent	Low	High
GlnC	Nitrogen excess	High	High	Low
GlnC	Nitrogen limited	High	High	Low

[a] The results are of several experiments with different strains grown in glucose-ammonia-glutamine medium (nitrogen excess) or glucose-limiting glutamine medium (nitrogen limiting). The Gln+ strain is a wild type control, the Gln− is a glutamine auxotroph lacking glutamine synthetase activity, and the GlnC produces high glutamine synthetase activity independent of the nitrogen source. The relative amounts of glutamine synthetase and histidase activities are recorded as being either low or high. The information is summarized from References 39, 40, and 41.

thetase also affected a separate factor involved in control, the evidence for glutamine synthetase itself being that the control element came from further genetic and biochemical studies.[42-46] Genetic studies of mutations in or near the structural gene for glutamine synthetase (*glnA*) in *K. aerogenes* placed mutations affecting both the regulation and activity of glutamine synthetase within the same gene. The majority of mutants analyzed were of three types. One type caused the loss of glutamine synthetase activity, a second caused elevated production of glutamine synthetase, and a third caused elevated production of an immunologically reacting, but enzymologically inactive, glutamine synthetase protein.[44,45] The placement of these mutations, particularly those of the third class, within the *glnA* gene, was particularly important. Because the mutations within *glnA* altered glutamine synthetase activity, while simultaneously affecting the regulation of histidase, glutamate dehydrogenase, and glutamine synthetase, it was proposed that glutamine synthetase was the regulatory molecule that mediated these effects.

With these results as a basis, it was proposed that glutamine synthetase was a regulatory protein (Figure 2). Its involvement as a positive regulator of histidase synthesis was extended to other enzymes involved in nitrogen utilization and placed glutamine synthetase as a key component for general nitrogen control or nitrogen catabolite repression.[35] Although the finding that glutamate dehydrogenase activities decreased when glutamine synthetase activities increased was not as extensively investigated, it was suggested that glutamine synthetase functioned as a negative effector to decrease its synthesis.[41,47] In addition, the demonstration that mutations within *glnA* caused elevated production of the glutamine synthetase protein implicated glutamine synthetase as a component in its own regulation.[45] This led to the model that glutamine synthetase is autogenously controlled (see Figure 2). Thus, there were two separate functions for glutamine synthetase as a regulatory molecule; one as a nitrogen control element and the other as a component in its own regulation.

The only direct biochemical test of either model of regulation used a purified transcription system to examine the regulation of the *hut* genes in vitro.[48] The transcription of *hut* specific mRNA was reported to be dependent on the addition of certain factors. Because *hut* expression is dependent on cyclic AMP and the cyclic AMP binding protein (CAP) when histidine is used as a carbon source, it was expected that these components would stimulate *hut* mRNA

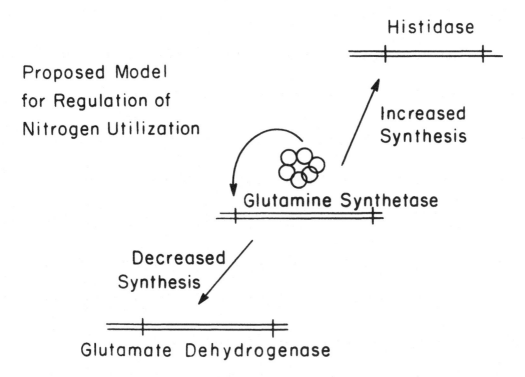

FIGURE 2. Diagram of the model for glutamine synthetase as a regulatory protein. The arrow to histidase illustrates the concept that glutamine synthetase functioned as a positive effector for increasing synthesis of histidase and other nitrogen utilization proteins. The arrow down to glutamate dehydrogenase represents the decreased synthesis of the enzyme whenever glutamine synthetase activities were elevated. The arrow for glutamine synthetase illustrates the proposal that glutamine synthetase is involved in the control of its own synthesis.

synthesis. The results showed that *hut* mRNA increased eight fold when cyclic AMP and CAP were included in the reaction mixture. When cyclic AMP and CAP were omitted and purified nonadenylylated glutamine synthetase added, the production of *hut* mRNA was again stimulated.[48] An important control in this experiment was the demonstration that the adenylylated form of glutamine synthetase did not activate transcription. These results focused attention on the nonadenylylated form of glutamine synthetase as an activator which stimulated transcription of *hut* and other nitrogen utilization genes.

Another result used to support the model was the finding that the glutamine synthetase protein binds DNA.[49] Biochemical experiments showed that glutamine synthetase binds DNA in crude extracts, and it can be sedimented with the DNA by centrifugation or polyethylene glycol precipitation.[49] When purified glutamine synthetase was mixed with DNA and examined under an electron microscope, complexes between the protein and DNA were found. These experiments demonstrated a general affinity of glutamine synthetase for DNA, but a specific binding to DNA control regions could not be demonstrated.[35] The lack of specificity could be explained by the inability to reproduce the exact conditions necessary for binding during the in vitro experiments or by the absence of another factor critical to the binding. The results of more recent experiments, to be discussed below, have shown that other factors are involved in the control of nitrogen utilization. Because of the importance of the in vitro experiments for testing the factors necessary for regulation, a critical examination of the activation of *hut* transcription is in progress and should help identify the necessary components.[50]

For the purposes of this discussion on glutamine synthetase as a multifunctional protein, the finding that the enzyme has an affinity for DNA is interesting. Such an affinity would

Table 2
SUMMARY OF GENES WITH PRODUCTS INVOLVED IN GLUTAMINE
SYNTHETASE AND/OR NITROGEN UTILIZATION REGULATION

Gene	Other designation	Genetic information	Comment
glnA	—	—	Gene for glutamine synthetase
glnB[39]	—	Not co-transducible with *glnA*	Gene for PII protein
glnF [54-57]	*ntrA*[59]	Not co-transducible with *glnA*	Unknown product needed for gluta- mine synthetase expression
glnG[57]	*ntrC*;[59] *glnR*[58]	Co-transducible with *glnA*	Unknown product involved in gluta- mine synthetase regulation
glnL[60,61]	*ntrB*[59]	Co-transducible with *glnA*	Unknown product involved in gluta- mine synthetase regulation

be expected if glutamine synthetase is to function as a regulatory protein, in which DNA binding is critical, and binding to DNA would establish a new biochemical function for the glutamine synthetase protein. From this viewpoint, the biochemical experiments necessary to directly determine whether glutamine synthetase has a specific affinity for DNA binding are extremely important and need to be reexamined.

B. Components to Be Added to the Early Model

The above information has surveyed a few of the primary reports leading to the model illustrated in Figure 2. The following portion will briefly outline data showing the existence of other factors that need to be incorporated into the model.

The first glutamine auxotroph reported had a mutation that was not within the glutamine synthetase structural gene of *K. aerogenes*.[39] The reversion of this strain to glutamine prototrophy yielded mutants with mutations near or within *glnA* that caused elevated expression of glutamine synthetase. These results implied that the original mutations causing auxotrophy were in a gene whose product was necessary for the production of glutamine synthetase. This gene was designated *glnB* and reported to encode a regulatory protein for glutamine synthetase.[39] Later, the *glnB* product was identified as being the PII protein, which determines whether the adenyl transferase adenylylates or deadenylylates glutamine synthetase, and its involvement in regulation was thought to function indirectly through the adenylylated glutamine synthetase.[51] Since recent reports suggest that the elimination of the PII protein product leads to elevated synthesis of glutamine synthetase, the mechanism by which the *glnB* product participates in influencing glutamine synthetase production is not clear.[52,53]

The existence of genes other than the structural gene, *glnA* or *glnB*, that function in regulation have been described. The first demonstration of another regulatory component was from Kustu's laboratory,[54] where she and her co-workers obtained glutamine auxotrophs of *S. typhimurium* with mutations unlinked by transduction to either *glnA* or *glnB*. This gene, *glnF*, was later shown to exist in *K. aerogenes*, *K. pneumoniae*, and *E. coli*.[55-57] The product of the *glnF* gene is not known, but it is presumably needed as a positive factor for the expression of both glutamine synthetase and other nitrogen utilization genes.

Revertants of strains with *glnF* mutations often have second site mutations linked with the *glnA* gene. These mutations were clearly shown to lie in a gene separate from *glnA* in both *S. typhimurium*, where this gene was called *glnR*, and *E. coli* where this gene was called *glnG*.[57,58] Recent work has shown that at least one other gene near *glnA* exists that is involved in regulation (Table 2).[59-61]

Although models have been proposed for the functions of these gene products and many others can be considered, none have been tested. Thus, for the purposes of this chapter, the discussion of these genes and their possible products will be limited to the view of how they affect the possibility of glutamine synthetase as a multifunctional protein involved in regulation. The primary consideration is that the existence of these genes must be incorporated into the model for glutamine synthetase and nitrogen utilization regulation. Their existence also complicates the interpretation of the earlier work that led to the original model.

C. Discussion of Current Information

Because the in vitro transcription experiments with the *hut* operon provided the best direct evidence for the model, the identification of new factors presumably important during transcription makes a reappraisal of those results necessary. One method to reconcile these findings would be to suggest that the glutamine synthetase used in the in vitro experiments contained some of these factors as contaminating proteins and that their presence was responsible for the stimulation of *hut* mRNA transcription. If these proteins were present, it may be that they co-purified with glutamine synthetase as a complex. The genetic data have so far been useful for showing that new gene products are involved in regulation. The investigations have not yet identified the products nor explained how they function. Given the diversity of the metabolic junction we are considering and the lack of information on the functions of these components, it seems premature to eliminate the possibility of several proteins, including glutamine synthetase, functioning as a complex. Another consideration is that these investigations have been designed to identify the major factors responsible for large changes in enzyme levels; investigations of factors involved in subtle changes or in control during growth transitions have not been identified. Although these smaller changes may be more difficult to test with in vitro transcription experiments, these investigations will be important for more precisely determining whether glutamine synthetase functions with the other factors in regulation.

The other results that caused a reevaluation of the model was the demonstration that genes exist near *glnA* that are involved in regulation. Their presence poses the question of whether the original mutations in *K. aerogenes* that affected regulation lie in these genes rather than in *glnA*. Significant to this consideration is the finding that the fusion of the gene for β-galactosidase to the *glnA* control region gives a strain with β-galactosidase regulation that mimics that of glutamine synthetase, even in the absence of a glutamine synthetase. Although these results imply that the glutamine synthetase protein is not necessary for regulation, not all features have been examined.[62] Clearly, the regulation of both glutamine synthetase and nitrogen utilization are complicated processes involving a variety of components. These components need to be added to the proposed models, but the question of whether the proposal that glutamine synthetase is a regulatory protein must be totally discarded is extremely difficult to answer.

Despite the ability to explain many aspects of glutamine synthetase and nitrogen utilization regulation without including glutamine synthetase, there remain a number of results implicating glutamine synthetase in some aspect of regulation. For example, temperature-sensitive glutamine auxotrophs of *S. typhimurium* have been isolated that fail to make *glnA* specific mRNA at the restrictive temperature.[63,64] The mutations affecting the transcription of *glnA* mRNA lie in the *glnA* gene and alter the stability of glutamine synthetase. The properties of these mutants are consistent with the model that mutations within *glnA* can alter glutamine synthetase regulation.

One mechanism that may reconcile some apparently conflicting genetic results would suggest that transcription of the *glnA* gene may continue into the adjacent regulatory genes (*glnL* and *glnG*) under certain circumstances.[65,66] If transcription continues from the *glnA* gene into these regulatory genes, then some mutations within *glnA* could have a polar effect on the transcription of downstream genes. As a consequence, synthesis of the regulatory products would be decreased, causing the control of glutamine synthetase and nitrogen utilization to be altered. We have determined the DNA sequence for the junction between *glnA* and the downstream genes of *S. typhimurium* and have found a sequence that could encode four glutamines if translated.[29] Although this region differs from that found for attenuators of other biosynthetic operons, it is tempting to speculate that this section may modulate transcription from *glnA* into the downstream gene. This sequence is followed by an idealized Pribnow heptamer and a possible translation start for a new protein. If transcription can also start at the Pribnow heptamer, then synthesis of the protein from this first regulatory gene could occur at a basal level. When a cell is limited for glutamine, then continued transcription from the *glnA* gene, through the region with the four glutamine codons, and into the regulatory gene it would increase synthesis of this gene product. This would effectively increase the expression of the regulatory gene during glutamine limitation. The consequences of this increased expression would be to change the regulation of glutamine synthetase as well as other nitrogen utilization genes. Experiments are in progress to characterize this region and to determine if continued transcription ever occurs from the *glnA* gene through the intergenic region and into the downstream gene. If such a mechanism occurs, then it is possible that mutations within *glnA* do in fact alter regulation, but it is the mutation itself, rather than the glutamine synthetase, that is crucial.

V. CONCLUDING REMARKS

Our perception of the complexity of nitrogen metabolism has expanded considerably during the last few years. The current features of the control are too unwieldy to predict all the components and their functions that are needed to produce the extensive modulation of the protein levels that are observed. However, the combination of the mutant studies with the detailed information provided by DNA sequencing should help simplify the current picture during the next few years.

Even though the question of whether glutamine synthetase is a regulatory protein with an affinity for DNA binding or for associations with other proteins remains unresolved. Glutamine synthetase clearly remains a fascinating protein. Its large, complex structure has numerous sites for small molecules, such as metal ions, substrates, and feedback inhibitors. In addition, the protein is a substrate for the enzyme adenyl transferase, which can covalently attach an AMP moiety to each subunit. Thus, independent of whether glutamine synthetase also functions alone or in a complex with other components as a regulatory protein, it has a multitude of exciting biochemical features.

ACKNOWLEDGMENTS

The preparation of this article was supported by Public Health Service Grant GM25251 from the National Institute of General Medical Sciences, by a Grant PCM23248 from the National Science Foundation, and by Research Career Development Award GM00449 from the National Institute of General Medical Sciences.

REFERENCES

1. **Krebs, H. A.,** Metabolism of amino acids. IV. The synthesis of glutamine from glutamic acid and ammonia, and the enzymic hydrolysis of glutamine in animal tissues, *Biochem. J.*, 29, 1951, 1935.
2. **Prusiner, S. and Stadtman, E. R.,** *The Enzymes of Glutamine Metabolism*, Academic Press, New York, 1973.

3. **Mora, J. and Palacios, R.**, *Glutamine: Metabolism, Enzymology and Regulation,* Academic Press, New York, 1980.

4. **Stadtman, E., Ginsburg, A., Ciardi, J., Yeh, J., Hennig, S., and Shapiro, B.**, Multiple molecular forms of glutamine synthetase produced by enzyme catalyzed adenylylation and deadenylylation reactions, *Adv. Enzyme Reg.,* 8, 99, 1970.

5. **Ginsburg, A. and Stadtman, E.**, Regulation of glutamine synthetase in *Escherichia coli,* in *The Enzymes of Glutamine Metabolism,* Prusiner, S. and Stadtman E. R., Eds., Academic Press, New York, 1973, 9.

6. **Stadtman, E. and Ginsburg, A.**, The glutamine synthetase of *Escherichia coli:* structure and control, in *The Enzymes,* Vol. 10, 3rd ed., Boyer, P. D., Ed., Academic Press, New York, 1974, 755.

7. **Meister, A.**, Catalytic mechanism of glutamine synthetase; overview of glutamine metabolism, in *Glutamine: Metabolism, Enzymology, and Regulation,* Mora, J. and Palacios, R., Eds., Academic Press, New York, 1980, chap. 1.

8. **Bender, R. and Streicher, S.**, Glutamine synthetase regulation, adenylylation state, and strain specificity analyzed by polyacrylamide gel electrophoresis, *J. Bacteriol.,* 137, 1000, 1979.

9. **Valentine, R. C., Shapiro, B. M., and Stadtman, E. R.**, Regulation of glutamine synthetase. XII. Electron microscopy of the enzyme from *Escherichia coli, Biochemistry,* 7, 2143, 1968.

10. **Miller, R., Shelton, E., and Stadtman, E.**, Zinc-induced paracrystalline aggregation of glutamine synthetase, *Arch. Biochem. Biophys.,* 163, 155, 1974.

11. **Frey, T. G., Eisenberg, D., and Eiserling, F. A.**, Glutamine synthetase forms three- and seven-stranded helical cables, *Proc. Natl. Acad. Sci. U.S.A.,* 72, 3402, 1975.

12. **Ronzio, R. A. and Meister, A.**, Phosphorylation of methionine sulfoximine by glutamine synthetase, *Proc. Natl. Acad. Sci. U.S.A.,* 59, 164, 1968.

13. **Gass, J. D. and Meister, A.**, Computer analysis of the active site of glutamine synthetase, *Biochemistry,* 9, 1380, 1970.

14. **Rowe, W. B. and Meister, A.**, Studies on the inhibition of glutamine synthetase by methionine sulfone, *Biochemistry,* 12, 1578, 1973.

15. **Tate, S. S. and Meister, A.**, Glutamine synthetases of mammalian liver and brain, in *The Enzymes of Glutamine Metabolism,* Prosiner, S. and Stadtman, E. R., Eds., Academic Press, New York, 1973, 77.

16. **Wedler, F.**, Mechanisms of substrate binding with glutamine synthetase, *J. Biol. Chem.,* 249, 5080, 1974.

17. **Wedler, F. C. and Horn, B. R.**, Catalytic mechanisms of glutamine synthetase enzymes, *J. Biol. Chem.,* 251, 7530, 1976.

18. **Hunt, J. B. and Ginsburg, A.**, Mn^{2+} and substrate interactions with glutamine synthetase from *Escherichia coli, J. Biol. Chem.,* 255, 590, 1980.

19. **Shrake, A., Whitley, E., Jr., and Ginsburg, A.**, Conformational differences between unadenylylated and adenylylated glutamine synthetase from *Escherichia coli* on binding L-methionine sulfoximine, *J. Biol. Chem.,* 255, 581, 1980.

20. **Balakrishnan, M., Villafranca, J., and Brenchley, J.**, Glutamine synthetase from *Salmonella typhimurium.* Manganese (II), substrate and inhibitor interaction with the unadenylylated enzyme, *Arch. Biochem. Biophys.,* 181, 603, 1977.

21. **Villafranca, J. J., Ash, D. E., and Wedler, F. C.**, Evidence for methionine sulfoximine as a transition-state analog for glutamine synthetase from NMR and EPR data, *Biochem. Biophys. Res. Commun.,* 66, 1003, 1975.

22. **Miller, E. and Brenchley, J.**, Mutations linked to the glutamine synthetase structural gene affecting nitrogen metabolism in *Salmonella typhimurium,* in *Abstr. Ann. Mtg. Am. Soc. Microbiol.,* 1979, K118.

23. **Miller, E. S. and Brenchley, J. E.**, L-Methionine-SR-sulfoximine resistant glutamine synthetase from mutants of *Salmonella typhimurium, J. Biol. Chem.,* 256, 11307, 1982.

24. **Heinrikson, R. L. and Kingdon, H. S.**, Primary structure of *Escherichia coli* glutamine synthetase. II. The complete amino acid sequence of a tryptic heneicosapeptide containing covalently bound adenylic acid, *J. Biol. Chem.,* 246, 1099, 1971.

25. **Hohman, R. J. and Stadtman, E. R.**, Use of AMP specific antibodies to differentiate between adenylylated and unadenylylated *E. coli* glutamine synthetase, *Biochem. Biophys. Res. Commun.,* 82, 865, 1978.

26. **Lei, M., Aebi, U., Heidner, E. G., and Eisenberg, D.**, Limited proteolysis of glutamine synthetase is inhibited by glutamate and by feedback inhibitors, *J. Biol. Chem.,* 254, 3129, 1979.

27. **Dautry-Varsat, A., Cohen, G. N., and Stadtman, E. R.**, Some properties of *Escherichia coli* glutamine synthetase after limited proteolysis by subtilism, *J. Biol. Chem.,* 254, 3124, 1979.

28. **Koduri, R. K., Bedwell, D. M., and Brenchley, J. E.**, Characterization of a *Hind*III-generated fragment carrying the glutamine synthetase gene of *Salmonella typhimurium, Gene,* 11, 227, 1980.

29. **Koduri, R., Ho, N., and Brenchley, J. E.**, manuscript in preparation, 1981.

30. **Kingdon, H. S.**, personal communication, 1980.

31. **Villafrance, J. J., Rhee, S. G., and Chock, P. B.,** Topographical analysis of regulatory and metal ion binding sites on glutamine synthetase from *Escherichia coli:* ^{13}C and ^{31}P nuclear magnetic resonance and fluorescence energy transfer study, *Proc. Natl. Acad. Sci. U.S.A.,* 75, 1255, 1978.

32. **Frink, R. J., Eisenberg, D., and Glitz, D. G.,** Localization of the site of adenylylation of glutamine synthetase by electron microscopy of an enzyme-antibody complex, *Proc. Natl. Acad. Sci. U.S.A.,* 75, 5778, 1979.

33. **Holman, R. J. and Stadtman, E. R.,** Use of AMP specific antibodies to differentiate between adenylylated and unadenylylated *E. coli* glutamine synthetase, *Biochem. Biophys. Res. Commun.,* 82, 865, 1978.

34. **Kirschner, K. and Bisswanger, H.,** Multifunctional proteins, *Ann. Rev. Biochem.,* 45, 143, 1976.

35. **Tyler, B.,** Regulation of the assimilation of nitrogen compounds, *Ann. Rev. Biochem.,* 47, 1127, 1978.

36. **Magasanik, B., Lund, P., Neidhardt, F. C., and Schwartz, D. T.,** Induction and repression of the histidine-degrading enzymes in *Aerobacter aerogenes, J. Biol. Chem.,* 240, 4320, 1965.

37. **Neidhardt, F. C. and Magasanik, B.,** Reversal of the glucose inhibition of histidase biosynthesis in *Aerobacter aerogenes, J. Bacteriol.,* 73, 253, 1957.

38. **Prival, M. and Magasanik, B.,** Resistance to catabolite repression of histidase and proline oxidase during nitrogen limited growth of *Klebsiella aerogenes, J. Biol. Chem.,* 246, 6288, 1971.

39. **Prival, M., Brenchley, J., and Magasanik, B.,** Glutamine synthetase and the regulation of histidase formation in *Klebsiella aerogenes, J. Biol. Chem.,* 248, 4334, 1973.

40. **Brenchley, J., Prival, M., and Magasanik, B.,** Regulation of the synthesis of enzymes responsible for glutamate formation in *Klebsiella aerogenes, J. Biol. Chem.,* 248, 6122, 1973.

41. **Magasanik, B., Prival, M. J., and Brenchley, J. E.,** Glutamine synthetase, regulator of the synthesis of glutamate forming enzymes, in *The Enzymes of Glutamine Metabolism,* Prusiner, S. and Stadtman, E., Eds., Academic Press, New York, 1973, 65.

42. **Streicher, S., Bender, R., and Magasanik, B.,** Genetic control of glutamine synthetase in *Klebsiella aerogenes, J. Bacteriol.,* 121, 320, 1975.

43. **Deleo, A. and Magasanik, B.,** Identification of the structural gene for glutamine synthetase in *Klebsiella aerogenes, J. Bacteriol.,* 121, 313, 1975.

44. **Bender, R. A. and Magasanik, B.,** Regulatory mutations in the *Klebsiella aerogenes* structural gene for glutamine synthetase, *J. Bacteriol.,* 132, 100, 1977.

45. **Bender, R. A. and Magasanik, B.,** Autogenous regulation of the synthesis of glutamine synthetase in *Klebsiella aerogenes, J. Bacteriol.,* 132, 106, 1977.

46. **Bender, R., Janssen, K., Resnick, A., Blumenberg, M., Foor, F., and Magasanik, B.,** Biochemical parameters of glutamine synthetase from *Klebsiella aerogenes, J. Bacteriol.,* 129, 1001, 1977.

47. **Bender, R. A., Macabuso, A., and Magasanik, B.,** Glutamate dehydrogenase: genetic mapping and isolation of regulator mutants of *Klebsiella aerogenes, J. Bacteriol.,* 127, 141, 1976.

48. **Tyler, B., DeLeo, A., and Magasanik, B.,** Activation of transcription of *hut* DNA by glutamine synthetase, *Proc. Natl. Acad. Sci. U.S.A.,* 71, 225, 1974.

49. **Streicher, S. L. and Tyler, B.,** Purification of glutamine synthetase from a variety of bacteria, *J. Bacteriol.,* 142, 69, 1980.

50. **Boylan, S. A., Janssen, K. A., and Bender, R. A.,** In vitro transcription of *Klebsiella aerogenes* histidine utilization genes by the homologous RNA polymerase, in *Abstr. Ann. Mtg. Am. Soc. Microbiol.,* 1981, 136.

51. **Foor, F., Janssen, K., and Magasanik, B.,** Regulation of the synthesis of glutamine synthetase by adenylylated glutamine synthetase, *Proc. Natl. Acad. Sci. U.S.A.,* 72, 4844, 1975.

52. **Foor, F., Reuveny, Z., and Magasanik, B.,** Regulation of the synthesis of glutamine synthetase by the PII protein in *Klebsiella aerogenes, Proc. Natl. Acad. Sci. U.S.A.,* 77, 2636, 1980.

53. **Reuveny, Z., Foor, F., and Magasanik, B.,** Regulation of glutamine synthetase by regulatory protein PII in *Klebsiella aerogenes* mutants lacking adenylyltransferase, *J. Bacteriol.,* 146, 740, 1981.

54. **Garcia, E., Bancroft, S., Rhee, S. G., and Kustu, S.,** The product of a newly identified gene, *glnF,* is required for synthesis of glutamine synthetase in *Salmonella, Proc. Natl. Acad. Sci. U.S.A.,* 74, 1662, 1977.

55. **Gaillardin, C. and Magasanik, B.,** Involvement of the product of the *glnF* gene in the autogenous regulation of glutamine synthetase formation in *Klebsiella aerogenes, J. Bacteriol.,* 133, 1329, 1978.

56. **Leonards, J. and Goldberg, R.,** Regulation of nitrogen metabolism in glutamine auxotrophs of *Klebsiella pneumoniae, J. Bacteriol.,* 142, 99, 1980.

57. **Pahel, G. and Tyler, B.,** A new *glnA*-linked regulatory gene for glutamine synthetase in *Escherichia coli, Proc. Natl. Acad. Sci. U.S.A.,* 76, 4544, 1979.

58. **Kustu, S., Burton, D., Garcia, E., McCarter, L., and McFarland, N.,** Nitrogen control in *Salmonella:* regulation by the *glnR* and *glnF* gene products, *Proc. Natl. Acad. Sci. U.S.A.,* 76, 4576, 1979.

59. **McFarland, N., McCarter, L., Artz, S., and Kustu, S.,** Nitrogen regulatory locus *"glnR"* of enteric bacteria is composed of cistrons *ntrB* and *ntrC:* identification of their protein products, *Proc. Natl. Acad. Sci. U.S.A.,* 78, 2135, 1981.

60. **MacNeil, T., MacNeil, D., and Tyler, B.,** Fine-structure map of the *glnA-glnG* region in *Escherichia coli,* in *Abstr. Ann. Mtg. Am. Soc. Microbiol.,* 1981, 151.

61. **Roberts, G. P., MacNeil, T., Snyder, T., and Tyler, B.,** Identification and regulation of proteins encoded in the *glnA* region of *Escherichia coli,* in *Abstr. Ann. Mtg. Am. Soc. Microbiol.,* 1981, 151.

62. **Rothstein, D. M., Pahel, G., Tyler, B., and Magasanik, B.,** Regulation of expression from the *glnA* promoter of *Escherichia coli* in the absence of glutamine synthetase, *Proc. Natl. Acad. Sci. U.S.A.,* 77, 7372, 1980.

63. **Bedwell, D. M. and Brenchley, J. E.,** Temperature-sensitive glutamine auxotrophs of *Salmonella typhimurium,* in *Abstr. Ann. Mtg. Am. Soc. Microbiol.,* 1980, 199.

64. **Bedwell, D. and Brenchley, J.,** manuscript in preparation, 1981.

65. **Magasanik, B. and Rothstein, D. M.,** The role of glutamine synthetase in the regulation of bacterial nitrogen metabolism, in *Glutamine: Metabolism, Enzymology and Regulation,* Mora, J. and Palacios, R., Eds., Academic Press, New York, 1980, chap. 3.

66. **Tyler, B., Bloom, F., and Pahel, G.,** Regulation of nitrogen metabolism in *Escherichia coli,* in *Glutamine: Metabolism, Enzymology and Regulation,* Mora, J. and Palacios, R., Eds., Academic Press, New York, 1980, chap. 4.

INDEX

S